Facial Nerve Rehabilitation

Editor

DANIEL S. ALAM

FACIAL PLASTIC SURGERY CLINICS OF NORTH AMERICA

www.facialplastic.theclinics.com

Consulting Editor
J. REGAN THOMAS

February 2016 • Volume 24 • Number 1

ELSEVIER

1600 John F. Kennedy Boulevard • Suite 1800 • Philadelphia, Pennsylvania, 19103-2899

http://www.theclinics.com

FACIAL PLASTIC SURGERY CLINICS OF NORTH AMERICA Volume 24, Number 1
February 2016 ISSN 1064-7406, ISBN-13: 978-0-323-41686-3

Editor: Jessica McCool
Developmental Editor: Alison Swety

Facial Plastic Surgery Clinics of North America (ISSN 1064-7406) is published quarterly by Elsevier Inc., 360 Park Avenue South, New York, NY 10010-1710. Months of issue are February, May, August, and November. Business and Editorial Offices: 1600 John F. Kennedy Blvd., Suite 1800, Philadelphia, PA 19103-2899. Periodicals postage paid at New York, NY, and additional mailing offices. Subscription prices are $390.00 per year (US individuals), $575.00 per year (US institutions), $445.00 per year (Canadian individuals), $716.00 per year (Canadian institutions), $535.00 per year (foreign individuals), $716.00 per year (foreign institutions), $100.00 per year (US students), and $255.00 per year (foreign students). Foreign air speed delivery is included in all *Clinics* subscription prices. All prices are subject to change without notice. POSTMASTER: Send address changes to *Facial Plastic Surgery Clinics*, Elsevier Health Sciences Division, Subscription Customer Service, 3251 Riverport Lane, Maryland Heights, MO 63043. **Customer service: 1-800-654-2452 (US and Canada); 1-314-447-8871 (outside US and Canada); Fax: 314-447-8029; E-mail: journalscustomerservice-usa@elsevier.com (for print support); journalsonline support-usa@elsevier.com (for online support).**

Reprints. For copies of 100 or more of articles in this publication, please contact the Commercial Reprints Department, Elsevier Inc., 360 Park Avenue South, New York, NY 10010-1710. Tel.: 212-633-3874; Fax: 212-633-3820; E-mail: reprints@elsevier.com.

Facial Plastic Surgery Clinics of North America is covered in *MEDLINE/PubMed* (*Index Medicus*).

Contributors

CONSULTING EDITOR

J. REGAN THOMAS, MD, FACS
Professor and Chairman, Department of
Otolaryngology, University of Illinois at
Chicago, Chicago, Illinois

EDITOR

DANIEL S. ALAM, MD, FACS
The Queen's Head and Neck Institute, The
Queen's Medical Center; Professor of Surgery,
University of Hawaii, John A. Burns School of
Medicine, Honolulu, Hawaii

AUTHORS

DANIEL S. ALAM, MD, FACS
The Queen's Head and Neck Institute, The
Queen's Medical Center; Professor of Surgery,
University of Hawaii, John A. Burns School of
Medicine, Honolulu, Hawaii

BABAK AZIZZADEH, MD, FACS
Director, Center for Advanced Facial Plastic
Surgery, Beverly Hills, California; Associate
Clinical Professor of Surgery, Department of
Head and Neck Surgery, David Geffen School
of Medicine at UCLA, Los Angeles, California

KOFI D. OWUSU BOAHENE, MD
Associate Professor of Facial Plastic and
Reconstructive Surgery, Otolaryngology Head
and Neck Surgery, Department of
Otolaryngology Head and Neck Surgery, Johns
Hopkins University School of Medicine,
Baltimore, Maryland

JOHN J. CHI, MD
Assistant Professor, Division of Facial
Plastic and Reconstructive Surgery,
Washington University Facial Plastic
Surgery Center, Washington University
in St Louis–School of Medicine, St Louis,
Missouri

JACQUELINE DIELS, OT
University of Wisconsin Hospital and Clinics,
Madison, Wisconsin

JENNIFER KIM, MD
Associate Clinical Professor, Department of
Otolaryngology-Head and Neck Surgery,
University of Michigan Health System, Ann
Arbor, Michigan

**MORGAN LANGILLE, BSc (Hons), MD,
FRCS(C)**
Associate Professor, Department of Surgery,
Dalhousie University, Saint John, New
Brunswick, Canada

OMID B. MEHDIZADEH, MD
Resident, Otolaryngology/Head and Neck
Surgery, NYU Langone Medical Center, New
York, New York

KELLY J. PETTIJOHN, MD
Resident Surgeon, Department of
Head and Neck Surgery, David Geffen
School of Medicine at UCLA, Los Angeles,
California

PRABHJYOT SINGH, BSc, MD, MSc, FRCS(C)
Division of Otolaryngology-Head and Neck Surgery, Department of Surgery, The Scarborough Hospital, Toronto, Ontario

KALPESH VAKHARIA, MD, MS
Department of Otolaryngology Head and Neck Surgery, University of Maryland Medical School, Baltimore, Maryland

KAVITA VAKHARIA, MD, MS
Division of Plastic Surgery, Penn State Hershey Medical Center, Hershey, Pennsylvania

WILLIAM MATTHEW WHITE, MD
Director, Facial Plastic and Reconstructive Surgery, Otolaryngology/Head and Neck Surgery, NYU Langone Medical Center, New York, New York

Contents

> Bell's palsy is unilateral, acute onset facial paralysis that is a common condition. One in every 65 people experiences Bell's palsy in the course of their lifetime. The majority of patients afflicted with this idiopathic disorder recover facial function. Initial treatment involves oral corticosteroids, possible antiviral drugs, and protection of the eye from desiccation. A small subset of patients may be left with incomplete recovery, synkinesis, facial contracture, or hemifacial spasm. A combination of medical and surgical treatment options exist to treat the long-term sequelae of Bell's palsy.

> This article reviews the current literature supporting the use of botulinum toxin in producing symmetric facial features and reducing unwanted, involuntary movements. Methods, protocols, and adverse events are discussed. Additionally, the authors suggest that using botulinum toxin as therapy in postparalytic facial synkinesis can provide long-term results when used in conjunction with other treatment modalities.

> The preoperative assessment of the eye in facial paralysis is a critical component of surgical management. The degree of facial nerve paralysis, lacrimal secretion, corneal sensation, and lower eyelid position must be assessed accurately. Upper eyelid loading procedures are standard management of lagophthalmos. Lower eyelid tightening repositions the lower eyelid and helps maintain the aqueous tear film. Eyelid reanimation allows an aesthetic symmetry with blinking and restores protective functions vital to ocular preservation. Patients often have multiple nervous deficits, including corneal anesthesia. Other procedures include tarsorrhaphy, spring implantation, and temporalis muscle transposition; associated complications have rendered them nearly obsolete.

> Facial paralysis results from a variety of different causes. Patients with facial paralysis have cosmetic and functional defects that significantly affect quality of life. Surgical intervention has the potential to help improve cosmetic and functional outcomes. The two main categories of surgical rehabilitation are static and dynamic surgical procedures. Static rehabilitation of the midface is typically performed using autologous tissue grafts, allografts, synthetic grafts, permanent suspension sutures, and a novel technique using percutaneous suture–based slings.

Temporalis muscle tendon unit (MTU) transfer may be used as a single-stage procedure for dynamic reanimation of the paralyzed face. Principles and biomechanics of muscle function and tendon transposition are essential in optimizing outcome. Critical steps and pearls for success include minimizing scarring, maintaining glide plains, mobilizing adequate tendon length, insertion of MTU at ideal tension based on intraoperative dynamic tension-excursion relationship, and insertion of tendon as close to the lip margin as possible. Because muscles adapt to tension, load, and task changes by altering their sarcomere arrangement and muscle fiber composition, physiotherapy should be initiated to use the repurposed temporalis MTU for smile restoration.

The gracilis free flap is the ideal modality of emotive and spontaneous facial reanimation in patients with a viable contralateral facial nerve. A 2-stage procedure with a cross-face nerve graft followed by gracilis free flap inset is advocated. In this article, the anatomy of the gracilis muscle, alternative neural sources (including the masseteric nerve), and technical aspects of the procedure are discussed. The literature regarding outcomes and complications is reviewed.

This article discusses the use of the sternohyoid muscle for facial reanimation. The report outlines the rationale for use, the technical aspects of flap harvest, and early clinical outcomes. The utility of the flap and its comparative attributes relative to the gracilis flap are discussed.

 Videos of patients after neural reanimation surgery accompany this article

Facial paralysis can have a profound effect on the patient from both an aesthetic and functional point of view. Just as there are numerous etiologies of facial paresis, there are as many therapeutic options and variations of these options. This article reviews the most current surgical options for neural reanimation of a damaged facial nerve, including recent advances in nerve repair, conduit technology, and nerve transfers, as well as emerging technology in translational research with biomedical engineering and tissue engineering.

FACIAL PLASTIC SURGERY CLINICS OF NORTH AMERICA

THE CLINICS ARE AVAILABLE ONLINE!
Access your subscription at:
www.theclinics.com

Preface
Facial Paralysis: State of the Art

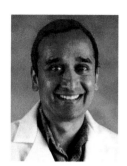

Daniel S. Alam, MD, FACS
Editor

Smiling is in many regards the most fundamental form of human communication. It is the simplest link from one person to another, a wordless spontaneous expression of the emotions that connect us to one another. The wonderful neural conduit that makes this and every other facial movement possible is the remarkable facial nerve. From protective functions like blinking, to the communication functions of our lips, to simple, subtle human expression, the facial nerve is the conductor of the symphony that is our face.

Because of its paramount importance, loss of function of this nerve is simply debilitating to those affected. Beyond the functional deficits, the psychological stigma of facial paralysis is daunting. Patients will often seek options far and wide to try to restore and rehabilitate their facial function. Therein lie both the rewards and the challenges that we face as physicians who care for these patients.

In some regards, no matter what approach we take, everything we do can potentially improve the lives of these patients. While this may seem a valid means to an end, we must not settle for the *simple* answer, and instead, we should seek the *best* one for the individual patient. The fact that so many potential solutions exist underlies the failings they all possess. The management of facial paralysis is inherently imperfect. Countless techniques exist because none is the Holy Grail.

Each offers its advantages and disadvantages, and all can be the "correct answer," but only in the "correct patient."

In this issue of *Facial Plastic Surgery Clinics of North America*, a collection of world class physicians provide insight into a single facet of the management of facial paralysis. As leaders in the field, they draw from their extensive clinical experience and expertise to provide a focused perspective on the problem. As stand-alone articles, none is the answer to every patient's needs; as a collection, we hope the issue will encompass the state of the art in the management of patients with facial paralysis. From medical management to complex microvascular techniques, the gamut of clinical options is covered.

I would like to thank the contributing authors for their valuable contributions to make this issue possible. More than any other arena of facial plastic surgery, the rehabilitation of the paralyzed face is littered with flawed solutions, and so, it's only in the gathering of minds that we will find our ultimate answers.

Daniel S. Alam, MD, FACS
The Queen's Head and Neck Institute
The Queen's Medical Center
1301 Punchbowl Avenue
Honolulu, HI 96813, USA

E-mail address:
dalam@queens.org

Facial Plast Surg Clin N Am 24 (2016) ix
http://dx.doi.org/10.1016/j.fsc.2015.10.001
1064-7406/16/$ – see front matter © 2016 Published by Elsevier Inc.

Bell's Palsy

Kavita Vakharia, MD, MS[a], Kalpesh Vakharia, MD, MS[b],*

KEYWORDS

- Bell's palsy • Facial paralysis • Herpes simplex virus (HSV) • Steroid • Anti-viral

KEY POINTS

- Bell's palsy describes an acute, unilateral facial paralysis believed to be caused by herpes simplex virus.
- It is most commonly found in people 15 to 45 years of age and occurs in 1 in 65 people in a lifetime.
- Medical treatment of Bell's palsy involves oral steroid and measures to protect the eye from desiccation.
- Most patients with Bell's palsy have spontaneous resolution.
- Patients who do not resolve completely may need further treatment to improve facial function, and manage secondary sequelae such as synkinesis, hypertonicity, or facial asymmetry.

INTRODUCTION

Accounts of facial paralysis date back to 5th century BCE by Hippocrates.[1] Sir Charles Bell described the anatomy of the facial nerve and its association with unilateral facial paralysis in 1821.[1] Since then, idiopathic facial paralysis has been termed Bell's palsy. Bell's palsy describes an acute, unilateral facial paralysis. This entity is a clinical diagnosis after exclusion of the other etiologies of facial paralysis through an astute patient history, physical examination, and laboratory or imaging studies if necessary. It is essential to understand that not all facial paralyses are Bell's palsy because a patient's management is driven by an identifiable etiology if one exists. Bell's palsy is defined by rapid onset, unilateral, lower motor neuron type of facial deficit, with lack of central nervous system, otologic, or cerebellopontine angle diseases. However, patients may have additional symptoms of hyperacusis, change in taste, facial sensation or pain, and epiphora. The facial paralysis can be partial or complete, although it is often self-limited. It can occur in women, children, and men; however, it is more common in people 15 to 45 years of age. Patients with compromised immune systems, diabetes, and those who are pregnant are at higher risk. The resulting facial paralysis can have devastating implications for a patient's function and appearance. Identification and management of patients to optimize return of facial function is crucial.

FACIAL NERVE ANATOMY

The complex anatomy of the facial nerve is relevant to understanding its function. In general, there are 3 portions of the facial nerve—the intracranial portion, the intratemporal portion, and the extratemporal portion. The facial nerve exits the brainstem at the cerebellopontine angle and enters the internal auditory canal of the temporal bone. In the internal auditory canal, it is accompanied by the VIIIth cranial nerve. Within the temporal bone there exist various segments of the nerve from the labyrinthine segment, the geniculate ganglion, tympanic segment and the vertical (mastoid) segment. Within the temporal bone, the first 3 branches are the greater superficial petrosal nerve, which provides secretomotor fibers to the lacrimal gland and conveys taste

[a] Division of Plastic Surgery, Penn State Hershey Medical Center, Hershey, PA, USA; [b] Department of Otolaryngology Head and Neck Surgery, University of Maryland Medical School, 419 West Redwood Street, Suite 370, Baltimore, MD 21201, USA
* Corresponding author.
E-mail addresses: kvakharia@smail.umaryland.edu; kalpesh.vakharia@gmail.com

Facial Plast Surg Clin N Am 24 (2016) 1–10
http://dx.doi.org/10.1016/j.fsc.2015.08.001
1064-7406/16/$ – see front matter © 2016 Elsevier Inc. All rights reserved.

from the soft palate; the nerve to the stapedius muscle, which is involved in dampening sound vibrations, and chorda tympani nerve, which conveys taste fibers from the anterior two-thirds of the tongue and supplies secretomotor fibers to the sublingual and submandibular glands. The nerve then exits the stylomastoid foramen and branches further in the extratemporal portion of it. The nerve gives off the posterior auricular nerve branch as well as branches to the posterior belly of the digastric and stylohyoid muscles. The main trunk of the facial nerve is found within the parotid gland, where it further divides into a frontozygomatic (upper) and cervicofacial (lower) division at the pes anserinus ("goose's foot). After that division the nerve divides into 5 major branches: the frontal, zygomatic, buccal, marginal mandibular, and cervical. These nerve branches go on to innervate the muscles of facial expression.

INCIDENCE

Bell's palsy is found fairly equally in males and females, but there tends to be a slightly greater occurrence in men older than 40 years old and in women younger than 20.[2] In general, the greatest incidence is seen in the 15- to 45-year-old age group.[3] In the general population, the incidence ranges from 11.5 to 40.2 per 100,000.[4] In the United States, the incidence ranges from 25 to 30 per 100,000, in Japan, it is reported as 30 per 100,000, and in the United Kingdom, and it is 20.2 per 100,000.[4] This disease affects approximately 1 in 65 people in a lifetime.[5] On presentation, 70% of patients with Bell's palsy have complete paralysis and 30% have incomplete paralysis.[3] Bell's palsy affects the right and left sides of the face fairly equally. Bilateral paralysis is rare and occurs in 0.3% of patients. A personal history of Bell's palsy is found in 9%, and a family history of Bell's palsy is found in 8% of patients.[2] There is a greater incidence of Bell's palsy in patients with diabetes, hypertension, immunocompromised status, after upper respiratory viral infection, and in pregnancy.[3] Most patients with Bell's palsy experience spontaneous resolution; 84% have near normal facial function and 71% resolve completely.[6] In patients with incomplete paralysis, 94% recover completely within 4 months of onset.[6] However, only 61% of patients with complete paralysis have complete recovery.[6] Those who do not recover may be left with persistent facial weakness, synkinesis, or facial contracture. Synkinesis is defined as unintentional movement of a segment of the face during volitional movement of another segment.

ETIOLOGY

Numerous etiologies have been proposed for Bell's palsy, such as autoimmune disorders, infections, ischemic insults, and hereditary.[7,8] The most generally accepted etiology, however, is that of the herpes simplex virus (HSV-1) inducing edema of the facial nerve that results in the facial dysfunction seen in patients with Bell's palsy. HSV-1 enters the body through mucocutaneous contact and has an affinity for peripheral nerves. The virus can lay dormant in the ganglia of peripheral nerves until it is reactivated. The DNA of HSV-1 along with varicella zoster has been identified in endoneural fluid in patients with Bell's palsy.[9,10] Histopathologic studies of temporal bones of patients with Bell's palsy have also shown infiltration of lymphocytes and associated demyelination or axonal degeneration surrounding the facial nerve.[11] Although the viral etiology of Bell's palsy is accepted, given the circumstantial evidence, the exact etiology still is considered to be unclear. Risk factors for the development of Bell's palsy have been identified, and include pregnancy, severe preeclampsia, diabetes, upper respiratory tract infections, and hypertension, as well as obesity.[12]

DIAGNOSIS

Bell's palsy is a clinical diagnosis and is largely one of exclusion. Patients present with a sudden onset of facial weakness that tends to be unilateral and rapidly progressive. The facial weakness tends to reach its peak within 72 hours. Patients may also have accompanied hyperacusis, change in facial sensation, neck or periauricular pain, or dysgeusia. In some patients, pain tends to precede palsy; patients may feel a sense of fullness of the ear or ear pain before manifesting facial weakness. However, if pain is significant and accompanies Bell's palsy, the patient is believed to have the diagnosis of Ramsey–Hunt syndrome, which is thought to be caused by varicella zoster infection. Additionally, with the loss of facial function, patients have incomplete eye closure, which can result in corneal exposure and desiccation. A Bell's phenomenon has been described as an upward rotation of the globe when patients attempt to close their eyes. This, however, is only present in 75% of the population (**Fig. 1**). Moreover, in Bell's palsy, the associated loss of the orbicularis oculi muscle function impairs the adequate handling of tears. Patients tend to have epiphora owing to an ineffective pump mechanism to spread the tear film, combined with irritation of the eye itself. With the

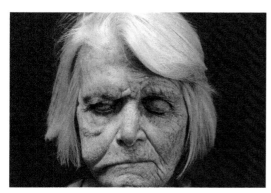

Fig. 1. A patient with facial paralysis demonstrating incomplete eye closure on the right side. She also demonstrates a Bell's phenomenon.

loss of facial muscular tone, the eyebrow along with the middle and lower face droop, giving patients the appearance that they have had a stroke. This can have a significant, negative impact on a person's self-image and the way they interact with others in society. Loss of function of the frontalis muscle results in immobility of the eyebrow and eventual brow ptosis that gives the impression of unhappiness and can limit one's visual field. Patients lose the ability to control their lips and mouth, thereby affecting their speech as well as their ability to eat and drink appropriately. Patients also may have trouble pronouncing certain words that have the letter *b* or *p* in them. Furthermore, they lose their ability to appropriately handle a food bolus, as well as saliva, thereby resulting in drooling or biting their own buccal mucosa. In addition to these functional deficits, patients with facial paralysis lose their ability to express themselves, such as with smiling. Consequently, the facial paralysis can have a significant negative impact on one's psychosocial well-being.

The differential diagnosis of facial paralysis is extensive and can be divided into broad categories of congenital, cerebrovascular, infectious, neoplastic, inflammatory or autoimmune, and traumatic. The clinician's history and physical examination is directed toward eliminating diseases within this differential diagnosis to diagnose a patient with Bell's palsy (**Box 1**).

FACIAL ASSESSMENT

Patients with Bell's palsy and the resulting facial dysfunction are assessed in terms of their severity. The face can be divided into various subunits and the disability in the various subunits has implications in the treatment options. The dominant subunits of the face are the forehead, periocular, nasal, cheek, perioral, and cervical regions. Facial paralysis can affect each of these subunits to a varying degree. Furthermore, synkinesis tends to affect multiple subunits upon facial movement. Synkinesis is the unintentional movement of a subset of facial muscles while performing intentional movement of another set of muscles.

There are numerous facial paralysis grading scales that have been described such as the Facial Nerve Grading Scale or the House–Brackmann (HB) scale[13,14] (**Table 1**). Each scale, if not well understood or used correctly, is subject to misinterpretation and inter-observer variability. The mostly widely accepted and used scale is the HB scale. This scale is used in clinical practice to describe patient's facial dysfunction, and provides a means to objectively monitor patients through treatment. Furthermore, the HB scale has been widely used in presenting facial dysfunction in research.

In addition to objective assessment via a facial paralysis grading scale, photo and video documentation are essential. A combination of photographs and videos can help providers and patients to document and monitor the extent of facial paralysis. Photograph views that should be taken include frontal, lateral, oblique, frontal view with brow elevation, eye closure, smiling, nasal snarl, puckering the lips, and showing one's teeth. These maneuvers highlight the facial function that is impaired as well as help to manifest any synkinesis that may be present.

DIAGNOSTIC TEST

Further diagnostic tests can be directed toward excluding other etiologies of facial paralysis. If risk factors for specific etiologies are identified during a complete history and physical examination, then laboratory testing as well as imaging should be directed toward supporting or excluding a particular etiology. For example, if Lyme disease is a possibility, then blood tests and analysis for antibodies to *Borrelia burgdorferi* should be performed. The American Academy of Otolaryngology—Head and Neck Surgery Foundation (AAO-HNSF) 2013 guidelines recommend against routine laboratory testing, unless the history and physical examination suggest an alternative diagnosis.[12]

CT scans with contrast of the face/neck and temporal bone or MRI with contrast of the face/neck and temporal bone can but used to evaluate the course of the facial nerve from the skull base into the face and the neck. MRI with contrast of patients with Bell's palsy has found enhancement along the facial nerve and often in the region of the

Box 1
Differential diagnosis of facial paralysis

Idiopathic
- Bell's palsy

Infectious
- HIV infection
- Lyme disease
- Poliomyelitis
- Meningitis/encephalitis
- Herpes
- Varicella zoster (Ramsay Hunt)
- Epstein–Barr virus
- Mumps
- Rubella
- Otitis media

Trauma
- Soft tissue trauma
- Temporal bone fracture
- Surgery
- Birth trauma
- Barotrauma

Autoimmune disease
- Guillain–Barre
- Melkersson–Rosenthal
- Multiple sclerosis
- Amyloidosis
- Sarcoidosis

Neoplasm – malignant, benign, primary, metastatic
- Acoustic neuroma
- Facial nerve tumor
- Neurofibroma
- Hemangioma
- Glomus tumor
- Parotid tumor
- Central nervous system tumor, that is, meningioma
- Head and neck cancer
- Squamous cell carcinoma
- Rhabdomyosarcoma
- Metastatic cancer (breast, lungs, kidney, colon, skin)

Congenital
- Mobius syndrome
- Congenital unilateral lower lip paresis
- Hemifacial macrosomia

- CHARGE (coloboma, heart defects, atresia of the choanae, retardation of growth and development, genital and urinary abnormalities, ear abnormalities and/or hearing loss)
- VACTERL (vertebral, anal atresia, cardiac, trachea, esophageal, renal, and limb defects)
- Chapple syndrome
- Branchiootorenal
- Nonsyndromic
- Mononeural agenesis
- Congenital absence of facial musculature
- Poland syndrome
- Thalidomide

Otologic
- Acute otitis media/mastoiditis
- Chronic otitis media
- Cholesteatoma

Intracranial
- Stroke

Data from Hohman MH, Hadlock TA. Etiology, diagnosis, and management of facial palsy: 2000 patients at a facial nerve center. Laryngoscope 2014;124:E283–93; and Adour KK, Hilsinger RL Jr, Callan EJ. Facial paralysis and Bell's palsy: a protocol for differential diagnosis. Am J Otol 1985;Suppl:68–3.

geniculate ganglion. The most common sites of enhancement tend to be the labyrinthine segment, and the distal meatal segment.[15,16] If a mass within the parotid is palpated then imaging with either CT scan with contrast or MRI with contrast should be undertaken. Initial presentation of Bell's palsy does not require imaging unless the history or physical suggests another diagnosis.

Table 1
House–Rackmann facial nerve grading system

Grade	Description	Characteristics
I	Normal	Normal facial function in all areas
II	Mild dysfunction	Gross: Slight weakness noticeable on close inspection; may have very slight synkinesis At rest: normal symmetry and tone Forehead motion: moderate to good function Eye motion: complete closure with minimum effort Mouth motion: slight asymmetry
III	Moderate dysfunction	Gross: obvious but not disfiguring difference between the two sides; noticeable but not severe synkinesis, contracture, or hemifacial spam At rest: normal symmetry and tone Motion: forehead - slight to moderate movement; eye – complete closure with effort; mouth - slight week with maximal effort
IV	Moderate to severe dysfunction	Gross: obvious weakness and/or disfiguring asymmetry At rest: normal symmetry and tone Motion: forehead – none; eye - incomplete closure; mouth – asymmetrical with maximal effort
V	Severe dysfunction	Gross: only barely perceptible motion At rest: asymmetry Motion: forehead – none; eye – incomplete closure, mouth – slight movement
VI	Total paralysis	No movement

Adapted from House JW, Brackmann DE. Facial nerve grading system. Otolaryngol Head Neck Surg 1985;93:146–7; with permission.

Furthermore, if patients fail to recover as expected, worsen, or show atypical features such as recurrence, segmental facial paralysis, and facial paralysis associated with other cranial nerve dysfunction, and there is no recovery after 3 months, imaging studies may be useful.[12]

For those patients who have complete facial paralysis, they may be considered for electrophysiological testing starting at 3 days after complete loss facial function. Electroneuronography involves transcutaneously stimulating the facial nerve and measuring the evoked compound muscle action potential via bipolar electrodes. If electroneuronography evaluation results in greater than 90% degeneration within the first 2 weeks, this tends to be a poor prognostic indicator and associated with incomplete recovery.[17] Additionally, if electromyography testing fails to show any evidence of neural regeneration, traditionally these patients were offered surgical decompression. However, given the lack of substantial evidence, surgical decompression is not offered universally to patients.

MANAGEMENT

The treatment of Bell's palsy involves early and late treatment based on the functional recovery and presence of any sequelae, such as synkinesis. In the early phase of treatment, management is directed toward improving facial recovery with interventions, such as steroids, antivirals, physical therapy, acupuncture, and protecting the eye during the period of facial dysfunction. The late phase of treatment is directed toward treating any residual facial movement deficit, and addressing synkinesis, facial contractures, or autonomic dysfunction such as crocodile tears or hemifacial spasm. Facial movement begins to return in patients with Bell's palsy approximately 3 weeks after onset of the paralysis.

Ocular protection is essential to protecting vision in both the short term and long term in patients with facial paralysis. Measures to prevent corneal exposure and desiccation include frequent application of artificial tears as well as lubrication combined with taping the eyelid shut at night. Consultation with an ophthalmologist is important to characterize any predisposing ocular diseases and assist with ocular protection. Clinicians should consider early eyelid weight implantation to help patients maximize ocular protection.

SURGICAL DECOMPRESSION

Because the understood pathophysiology of Bell's palsy is of nerve edema and associated nerve entrapment by the surrounding bony framework, this has led surgeons to advocate for surgical decompression. Surgical decompression involves removal of the bony surroundings of the nerve. The site of decompression of the nerve has changed over the years as an understanding of the site of the injury has been further defined. The first known case of decompression was reported in 1932 by Ballance. He advocated slitting the sheath in the descending segment of the nerve.[18] Since then, areas of decompression have ranged from anywhere from the meatus to the stylomastoid foramen. Surgeons have advocated a transmastoid approach to the facial nerve. A Cochrane review in 2014 of all literature as it relates to surgical management of Bell's palsy found only 2 randomized control trials from 1971. One of the trials found no statistically significant difference between surgical and nonoperative treatment and the second trial did not perform statistics; however, a significant difference was believed to be unlikely.[18]

The meatal foramen as well as the labyrinthine segment has been found to be the narrowest portion of the bony facial canal and the most common sites of nerve injury in Bell's palsy.[19–22] Based on this understanding, surgical decompression has been advocated via a middle fossa approach. If patients have greater than 90% degeneration on electroneuronography testing and no voluntary electromyography motor unit potentials, and present within 14 days of symptoms, they are considered surgical candidates. Gantz and colleagues[21] in their case-control series found that 91% of patients (n = 34) who were treated surgically achieved an HB I or HB II compared with 41% of patients (n = 36) who were treated with steroids alone. Other observational studies have reported similar findings ranging from 61% to 91% improvement to HB I or HB II.[22–24]

In 2013, the Academy of Otolaryngology clinical practice guideline committee made no recommendation either for or against surgical decompression for Bell's palsy. This lack of recommendation stems from the lack of strong evidence supporting or refuting surgical intervention especially because the surgical intervention has potential for serious side effects, such as hearing impairment and cerebrospinal fluid leak.[12] Currently, based on a lack of strong evidence, surgical decompression is not recommended as a standard approach to patients with Bell's palsy.

CORTICOSTEROID THERAPY

Because inflammation and edema of the facial nerve in patients with Bell's palsy has been well-documented, therapies directed toward addressing the inflammation remain the mainstay of therapy. Oral corticosteroids are believed to decrease inflammation and edema in the hopes of facilitating facial function recovery. Two very important, large, randomized clinical trials have found that oral corticosteroid treatment within 72 hours of onset of symptoms can have a clinically significant benefit on facial function recovery within patients with Bell's palsy.[25,26] Engstrom and colleagues[26] in 2008 found that prednisolone can significantly shorten the time to recovery in patients with Bell's palsy compared with treatment with placebo or valacyclovir alone or in combination. Sullivan and colleagues[25] in 2007 found that early treatment with prednisolone significantly improves the chance of complete recovery at 3 and 9 months. Both trials used prednisolone; however, the dosing schemes were slightly different. Engstrom and colleagues used 60 mg of prednisolone for 5 days and then reduced it by 10 mg/d for a total treatment time of 10 days. Sullivan and colleagues used 50 mg of prednisolone for 10 days. Based on these high-quality randomized controlled trials, the AAO-HNSF strongly recommends the administration of oral corticosteroids within 72 hours of onset of symptoms in patients that are greater than 16 years old.[12]

ANTIVIRAL THERAPY

As the pathophysiology of Bell's palsy is understood to be activation of HSV-1, clinicians have added antiviral therapy to the acute treatment of Bell's palsy. However, treatment with antiviral therapy has been very controversial. Patients have been treated with either valacyclovir or acyclovir. Clinicians have attempted to treat Bell's palsy with antiviral treatment alone or have added it to a regimen of corticosteroid therapy. Numerous researchers, through a combination of retrospective, observational, and randomized controlled trials, have attempted to determine if any benefit or harm from the addition of antiviral therapy exists. There were numerous conflicting results that have fed into the controversy and have left clinicians without a clear direction. The AAO-HNSF has recommended against oral antiviral monotherapy with new onset Bell's palsy based on high-quality randomized controlled trials. However, the guidelines leave the option to physicians of offering and providing oral antiviral therapy in addition to oral steroids within 72 hours of symptom onset based on randomized controlled trials with minor limitations in observational studies with equivalent benefit and harm.[12] Recent randomized control trials, as well as a 2015 Cochrane review, has found no benefit

from adding antivirals to corticosteroids in comparison with corticosteroids alone for patients with Bell's palsy. However, for patients with severe Bell's palsy as defined by HB scores of 5 and 6, there has been a demonstration of a reduction in the rate of incomplete recovery at 6 months when antivirals are combined with corticosteroids. Furthermore, there is no role for antivirals alone without corticosteroid administration.[27] Notably, pediatric Bell's palsy patients have not been included in the numerous antiviral trials; therefore, no evidence supporting use of antiviral therapy in pediatric patients exists.

PHYSICAL THERAPY

There has been much interest in physical therapy techniques for improvement of facial function after Bell's palsy. Interventions such as massage, facial exercises, biofeedback, thermal therapy, electrotherapy, and acupuncture have all been evaluated.[3,28] The most common type of physical therapy that has been advocated has been massage and facial exercises.[29–32] Although electrical stimulation has been evaluated in numerous studies, it has not been shown to be beneficial. Facial exercise has also been shown to show some improvement in moderate paralysis and chronic cases of facial paralysis.[29] Furthermore, it has been shown to decrease recovery time and sequelae in acute cases. Strong randomized control trials are still necessary, however, to continue supporting its use. Additionally, there needs to be higher quality trials to determine the efficacy of and role of acupuncture in chronic Bell's palsy cases.[33]

OUTCOMES

Fortunately, patients diagnosed with Bell's palsy tend to recover. Approximately 85% of patients experience some recovery in the first 3 weeks and the remaining 15% after 3 to 5 months[3]; 70% of all patients experience full recovery. Of the patients who do not recover, sequela was slight in 12% of patients, mild in 13%, and severe in 4%.[3] Treatment with steroids improves the rate of recovery to greater than 90%.[25] Numerous prognostic features have been evaluated such as age, gender, diabetes, hypertension, and extent of facial deficit at 1 week. Among these, the extent of facial deficit at 1 week correlated with level of nonrecovery.[34] If some level of recovery is not present then further diagnostic testing such as CT scan and MRI should be considered.

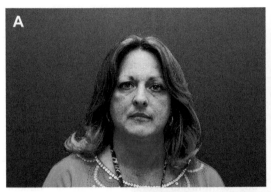
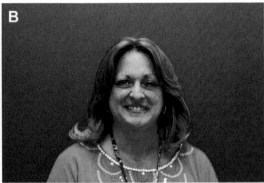
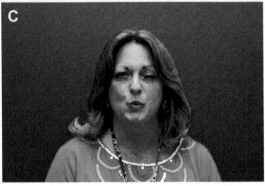

Fig. 2. A patient with synkinesis. (*A*) Face at rest. (*B*) Face with smile results in unintentional narrowing of left palpebral aperture. (*C*) Puckering results in near closure of left eye.

SYNKINESIS

Synkinesis is abnormal, involuntary facial muscle contraction during voluntary facial movement of a different group of facial muscles. This phenomenon is seen after recovery from facial nerve injury. The exact cause of synkinesis has not been characterized completely. The proposed mechanism is believed to be aberrant regeneration and sprouting of new facial nerve axons to facial muscular groups.[35–37] This aberrant innervation results in unintentional movement in one area of the face during intentional movement in another area of the face. For example, while smiling or laughing a patient may unintentionally close their eye; or during blink, the midface spasms (**Fig. 2**). Not only are these aberrant facial movements socially detrimental, patients complain of pain and facial tightness owing to these muscular spasms. The treatment of synkinesis involves biofeedback, physiotherapy, physical therapy, botulinum toxin injections, or surgery with selective neurectomy or myectomy or cross-face nerve grafting.[38–43]

LONG-TERM TREATMENT

Patients who achieve full functional recovery after Bell's palsy tend to not require any additional

treatment. However, the subgroups of patients that have incomplete recovery or secondary sequelae such as synkinesis, facial contracture, autonomic dysfunction, or hemifacial spasm require further treatment. Treatment tends to include a combination of physical therapy, chemodenervation with botulinum toxin, and periorbital procedures to correct brow ptosis or incomplete eye closure, along with static and dynamic techniques to achieve improved facial symmetry and, in some situations, dynamic facial reanimation. The various treatment options are discussed in additional detail elsewhere.

SUMMARY

Bell's palsy is a common cause of acute, unilateral facial paralysis. Although the exact etiology remains unclear, it is believed that HSV-1 virus mediates facial edema and consequently leads to facial paralysis. Fortunately, the majority of patients with Bell's palsy spontaneously recover facial function. Guidelines recommend initial treatment of patients with Bell's palsy with oral corticosteroids to improve facial function recovery. The addition of antiviral treatment is controversial, but recommended in severe cases where patients have complete loss of facial function. Surgical decompression as primary treatment of Bell's palsy has been controversial and is not currently recommend by published guidelines. A subgroup of patients may not recover completely and be left with long-term sequelae, such as facial contracture, asymmetry, autonomic dysfunction, hemifacial spasms, or synkinesis. A number of medical and surgical options are available to treat patients who have long-term sequelae from Bell's palsy.

REFERENCES

1. Sajadi MM, Sajadi MR, Tabatabaie SM. The history of facial palsy and spasm: Hippocrates to Razi. Neurology 2011;77:174–8.

2. Adour KK, Byl FM, Hilsinger RL Jr, et al. The true nature of Bell's palsy: analysis of 1,000 consecutive patients. Laryngoscope 1978;88:787–801.

3. Peitersen E. Bell's palsy: the spontaneous course of 2,500 peripheral facial nerve palsies of different etiologies. Acta Otolaryngol Suppl 2002;(549):4–30.

4. De Diego JI, Prim MP, Madero R, et al. Seasonal patterns of idiopathic facial paralysis: a 16-year study. Otolaryngol Head Neck Surg 1999;120:269–71.

5. Marson AG, Salinas R. Bell's palsy. West J Med 2000;173:266–8.

6. Peitersen E. The natural history of Bell's palsy. Am J Otol 1982;4:107–11.

7. Greco A, Gallo A, Fusconi M, et al. Bell's palsy and autoimmunity. Autoimmun Rev 2012;12:323–8.

8. Eviston TJ, Croxson GR, Kennedy PG, et al. Bell's palsy: aetiology, clinical features and multidisciplinary care. J Neurol Neurosurg Psychiatry 2015. [Epub ahead of print].

9. Murakami S, Mizobuchi M, Nakashiro Y, et al. Bell palsy and herpes simplex virus: identification of viral DNA in endoneurial fluid and muscle. Ann Intern Med 1996;124:27–30.

10. Furuta Y, Ohtani F, Sawa H, et al. Quantitation of varicella-zoster virus DNA in patients with Ramsay Hunt syndrome and zoster sine herpete. J Clin Microbiol 2001;39:2856–9.

11. Michaels L. Histopathological changes in the temporal bone in Bell's palsy. Acta Otolaryngol Suppl 1990;470:114–7 [discussion: 118].

12. Baugh RF, Basura GJ, Ishii LE, et al. Clinical practice guideline: Bell's palsy. Otolaryngol Head Neck Surg 2013;149:S1–27.

13. Ross BG, Fradet G, Nedzelski JM. Development of a sensitive clinical facial grading system. Otolaryngol Head Neck Surg 1996;114:380–6.

14. House JW, Brackmann DE. Facial nerve grading system. Otolaryngol Head Neck Surg 1985;93:146–7.

15. Nowak DA, Linder S, Topka H. Diagnostic relevance of transcranial magnetic and electric stimulation of the facial nerve in the management of facial palsy. Clin Neurophysiol 2005;116:2051–7.

16. Engstrom M, Thuomas KA, Naeser P, et al. Facial nerve enhancement in Bell's palsy demonstrated by different gadolinium-enhanced magnetic resonance imaging techniques. Arch Otolaryngol Head Neck Surg 1993;119:221–5.

17. May M, Blumenthal F, Klein SR. Acute Bell's palsy: prognostic value of evoked electromyography, maximal stimulation, and other electrical tests. Am J Otol 1983;5:1–7.

18. McAllister K, Walker D, Donnan PT, et al. Surgical interventions for the early management of Bell's palsy. Cochrane Database Syst Rev 2013;(10):CD007468.

19. Burmeister HP, Baltzer PA, Volk GF, et al. Evaluation of the early phase of Bell's palsy using 3 T MRI. Eur Arch Otorhinolaryngol 2011;268:1493–500.

20. Ge XX, Spector GJ. Labyrinthine segment and geniculate ganglion of facial nerve in fetal and adult human temporal bones. Ann Otol Rhinol Laryngol Suppl 1981;90:1–12.

21. Gantz BJ, Rubinstein JT, Gidley P, et al. Surgical management of Bell's palsy. Laryngoscope 1999;109:1177–88.

22. Fisch U. Surgery for Bell's palsy. Arch Otolaryngol 1981;107:1–11.

23. Yanagihara N, Hato N, Murakami S, et al. Transmastoid decompression as a treatment of Bell palsy. Otolaryngol Head Neck Surg 2001;124:282–6.

24. Friedman RA. The surgical management of Bell's palsy: a review. Am J Otol 2000;21:139–44.

25. Sullivan FM, Swan IR, Donnan PT, et al. Early treatment with prednisolone or acyclovir in Bell's palsy. N Engl J Med 2007;357:1598–607.

26. Engstrom M, Berg T, Stjernquist-Desatnik A, et al. Prednisolone and valaciclovir in Bell's palsy: a randomised, double-blind, placebo-controlled, multicentre trial. Lancet Neurol 2008;7:993–1000.

27. Gagyor I, Madhok VB, Daly F, et al. Antiviral treatment for Bell's palsy (idiopathic facial paralysis). Cochrane Database Syst Rev 2015;(7):CD001869.

28. Mosforth J, Taverner D. Physiotherapy for Bell's palsy. Br Med J 1958;2:675–7.

29. Beurskens CH, Heymans PG. Positive effects of mime therapy on sequelae of facial paralysis: stiffness, lip mobility, and social and physical aspects of facial disability. Otol Neurotol 2003;24:677–81.

30. Brach JS, VanSwearingen JM. Physical therapy for facial paralysis: a tailored treatment approach. Phys Ther 1999;79:397–404.

31. Ross B, Nedzelski JM, McLean JA. Efficacy of feedback training in long-standing facial nerve paresis. Laryngoscope 1991;101:744–50.

32. Segal B, Hunter T, Danys I, et al. Minimizing synkinesis during rehabilitation of the paralyzed face:

preliminary assessment of a new small-movement therapy. J Otolaryngol 1995;24:149–53.

33. Chen N, Zhou M, He L, et al. Acupuncture for Bell's palsy. Cochrane Database Syst Rev 2010;(8):CD002914.

34. Fujiwara T, Hato N, Gyo K, et al. Prognostic factors of Bell's palsy: prospective patient collected observational study. Eur Arch Otorhinolaryngol 2014;271: 1891–5.

35. Crumley RL. Mechanisms of synkinesis. Laryngoscope 1979;89:1847–54.

36. Chaco J. Misdirection of facial nerve fibers in Bell's palsy. ORL J Otorhinolaryngol Relat Spec 1974;36: 205–8.

37. Baker RS, Stava MW, Nelson KR, et al. Aberrant reinnervation of facial musculature in a subhuman primate: a correlative analysis of eyelid kinematics, muscle synkinesis, and motoneuron localization. Neurology 1994;44:2165–73.

38. VanSwearingen JM, Brach JS. Changes in facial movement and synkinesis with facial neuromuscular reeducation. Plast Reconstr Surg 2003;111:2370–5.

39. Nakamura K, Toda N, Sakamaki K, et al. Biofeedback rehabilitation for prevention of synkinesis after facial palsy. Otolaryngol Head Neck Surg 2003;128: 539–43.

40. Ito H, Ito H, Nakano S, et al. Low-dose subcutaneous injection of botulinum toxin type A for facial synkinesis and hyperlacrimation. Acta Neurol Scand 2007;115:271–4.

41. Guerrissi JO. Selective myectomy for postparetic facial synkinesis. Plast Reconstr Surg 1991;87: 459–66.

42. Zhang B, Yang C, Wang W, et al. Repair of ocular-oral synkinesis of postfacial paralysis using cross-facial nerve grafting. J Reconstr Microsurg 2010; 26:375–80.

43. Hohman MH, Lee LN, Hadlock TA. Two-step highly selective neurectomy for refractory periocular synkinesis. Laryngoscope 2013;123:1385–8.

Botulinum Toxin in the Treatment of Facial Paralysis

Omid B. Mehdizadeh, MD[a], Jacqueline Diels, OT[b],
William Matthew White, MD[c],*

KEYWORDS

• Synkinesis • Facial paralysis • Botulinum toxin • Asymmetry

KEY POINTS

• Combination treatment with neuromuscular retraining (NMR) exercises is essential for a better long-term outcome.
• A sequence of first evaluation and treatment with NMR is recommended. When resistant muscle groups are identified, treatment should be started with chemodenervation.
• Botulinum toxin can be injected in the affected synkinetic hemiface to relax hyperactive muscles and the normal hemiface for balance to restore facial symmetry.
• Challenging areas for treatment of synkinesis include the midface and lip depressor complex and should be addressed carefully.

INTRODUCTION

Synkinesis makes up the overwhelming majority of patients who present to a facial nerve center with facial movement disorders. The synkinetic facial movement can be subtle or completely disfiguring. Interestingly, patients who have synkinetic activity that is barely noticeable sometimes are the most disturbed by the condition. Most patients begin to see evidence of spastic activity of the facial muscles 6 months after recovery of their facial paralysis. Rarely, this can even occur in the early phase of recovery as well. Synkinetic activity should only occur on the hemifacial side of the original injury.

Restoration of permanent facial symmetry in the postparalyzed synkinetic face has been a mainstay of surgical treatment.[1–4] Myectomy, neurectomy, cross-face nerve grafts, and sling procedures have all been implemented in achieving outcomes. Although results can be satisfactory, they are invasive and irreversible. Botulinum toxin with and without neuromuscular therapy has shown promising utility as a nonoperative method in restoring normal facial features, with recent literature demonstrating increasingly long-term effects when used concurrently with neuromuscular training.[5–7]

Produced by various strains of *Clostridium botulinum*, multiple agents are currently available on the United States market. There are currently 4 pharmacologic forms in the United States, each with varying potencies and shelf lives: abobotulinumtoxinA (Dysport, Medicis Aesthetics, Inc, Scottsdale, AZ; Azzalure, Galderma Laboratories, Lausanne, Switzerland), incobotulinumtoxinA (Xeomin, Merz Aesthetics, Inc, Franksville, WI), onabotulinumtoxinA (Botox, Allergan, Inc, Irvine, C), and rimabotulinumtoxinB (Myobloc, Solstice Neurosciences, LLC, Louisville, KY).[8] Application remains percutaneous and intramuscular.

[a] NYU Langone Medical Center, 550 First Avenue - NBV 5E5, New York, NY 10016, USA; [b] Facial Nerve Clinic, UW Hospitals and Clinics, 600 Highland Avenue, Madison, WI 53792, USA; [c] NYU Ambulatory Care Center, 240 E 38th Street, 14th Floor, New York, NY 10016, USA
* Corresponding author.
E-mail address: William.white@nyumc.org

Facial Plast Surg Clin N Am 24 (2016) 11–20
http://dx.doi.org/10.1016/j.fsc.2015.09.008
1064-7406/16/$ – see front matter © 2016 Elsevier Inc. All rights reserved.

Pattern of injection into muscle groups, units administered, and frequency of treatment is not standardized. Amounts administered have varied from fractions of a unit per site[9] to hundreds in total,[5,10,11] with increasing risk of adverse events including oral incompetence, ptosis, diplopia, exposure keratopathy, malaise, and worsened cosmesis[10,12] with larger doses. These events are reversible, however, because the effects of the toxin diminish.

Botulinum toxin continues to expand from its first description in strabismus by Scott[13] in 1980 to its eventual approval by the US Food and Drug Administration for strabismus and blepharospasm in 1989. Additional benefits were recognized for aesthetic purposes by Carruthers and Carruthers[14] in their description of reduction in glabellar frown lines in 1992.

Those who endure the sequela of postparalytic synkinesis or abnormal involuntary facial movements have been shown to have diminished quality of life, social interactions, peripheral visual impairment, and a worsened self-impression of personal appearance. In many instances, botulinum toxin therapy has been shown to decrease the severity of these personal morbidities and improve quality of life[15] with validated methods of subjective assessment including the Facial Clinimetric Evaluation score,[16] Sunnybrook Facial Grading System,[17] and Synkinesis Assessment Questionnaire[18] currently in use.

Characterized by involuntary movement in the setting of volitional facial expressions, multiple patterns have been described after facial nerve injury including ocular, oral, and cervical synkinesias, dyskinesias, and hyperkesias. Typically, a patient might experience spasm of the eye with smiling or sometimes violent movements of the corner of the mouth with eye closure. Manifestations of various forms require personalized injection patterns to achieve optimal outcomes and aesthetics while minimizing side effects.[5] The toxin is typically administered to certain muscle groups that provide certain function (ie, eye closure or lip elevation) such as injection into the orbicularis oculi, corrugators, and frontalis muscles for upper synkinesias and zygomaticus, levator muscle of upper lip, orbicularis oris, depressor labii, depressor oris, and platysma muscles for lower division defects.[7,19] Functionally, botulinum toxin chemically dennervates the neuromuscular junction by permanently blocking presynaptic acetylcholine release at the synaptic junction.

Mention of botulinum toxin A as an alternate treatment of ocular synkinesia was first introduced by Putternam[20] in 1990. In his description of a single case report, he discusses a 28-year-old woman with "misdirection of the facial nerve" after Bell's Palsy causing ocular spasm with smiling.[20] Since then, the literature has been populated by numerous studies augmenting the role of botulinum toxin A in postparalytic facial synkinesia[5,9–12,15,21–29] evolving to hints of long-term improvement when used with concurrent neuromuscular training including half and whole face mirror feedback[6,7] and neuromuscular retraining (NMR) therapy.[26] The application of other traditional therapies in conjunction with botulinum toxin has yet to be elucidated.

Causes of postparalytic facial synkinesia are vast and varied, providing a universal platform for this minimally invasive therapy. Central iatrogenic tumor resections in the setting of vestibular and facial schwannomas,[27] middle ear surgery,[24] as well as peripheral parotid malignancies have been described.[27] Bells palsy and Ramsey Hunt syndrome have also been implicated,[9,19,27] in addition to traumatic skull base injury.[9]

The neurophysiology of these involuntary movements has yet to be fully understood. Aberrant peripheral facial nerve regeneration is most commonly attributed.[30–32] However, studies in the generation of synkinesis have demonstrated predictable patterns of regeneration thought to be owing to increased excitability within the facial nucleus itself.[33]

This article reviews the current literature supporting the use of botulinum toxin in producing symmetric facial features and reducing unwanted, involuntary movements. Methods, protocols, and adverse events are discussed. Additionally, the authors suggest that using botulinum toxin A therapy in postparalytic facial synkinesis can provide long-term results when used in conjunction with other treatment modalities.

EVALUATION

Before beginning therapy, a patient should undergo a thorough evaluation of their history of facial paralysis and a complete evaluation of their facial movements. Standardized photography and video recording should be performed to clearly document treatment efficacy. The 9 standard views include face at rest, brow elevation, complete eye closure, nose wrinkling, grin, full smile, pucker, whistle, and lower lip depression.

It is important during the evaluation to identify the "triggers" for eliciting the synkinesis. This most commonly is forceful eye closure or a puckering movement of the lips. Critical to the evaluation, the patient should be questioned their main concerns are and what areas of the face and neck are the most troubling. Patients typically remark about the discomfort of spasms around the eye or neck. Ideally, these areas should be addressed first and foremost. It is recommended to wait at least 6 months after the onset of facial paralysis to allow recovery. Any intervention before that time can potentially make the synkinesis worse.

Ideally, the patient should have an initial treatment by a physical or occupational therapist who has specific training in facial NMR. It is helpful for the physician to evaluate the patient before beginning therapy, which can help to determine the progress of treatment. A team approach can be very helpful to the patient.

THERAPEUTIC OPTIONS
Neuromuscular Retraining

Facial NMR is a specific subset of occupational and physical therapy developed for improving motor learning and functional outcomes in patients with facial paralysis, paresis and/or synkinesis after facial nerve injury. Facial NMR techniques are based on characteristics unique to the facial nerve and muscles it innervates (eg, lack of muscle spindles and presence of emotional, as well as volitional, neural inputs).[34] Facial NMR should not be confused with the more common, nonspecific therapies that promote gross motor, maximum effort exercises and electrical stimulation, both of which are contraindicated in facial paralysis.[35] Rather, NMR focuses on providing sensory information to enhance neural adaptation and learning via the practice of minimal, precisely coordinated movement patterns in conjunction with modalities such as surface electromyographic, proprioceptive, and mirror feedback. This comprehensive clinical program was first described by Balliet and colleagues[36] in 1982, who reported improved function in patients more than 2 years after facial nerve injury. Acquisition of new motor behaviors was attributed to brain plasticity, the capacity of the central nervous system to modify its organization, resulting in lasting functional change.[36]

From a nonoperative rehabilitation perspective, facial muscles play a different role than other muscles in the body. Simply stated, their purpose is to move the facial skin in various directions, producing a wide variety of expressions used primarily for nonverbal communication, eye closure, and oral motor functions. The subtleties of human expression require a delicate balance of activity among multiple facial muscles. The presence of synkinesis destroys the normal balance.

Synkinesis is the most common condition treated by the facial NMR therapist. Because it does not occur in other areas of the body, there is no precedent for identifying and understanding it. When muscles contract out of sequence, the facial skin is displaced in an unusual direction, creating a distorted expression. What seems to be lack of movement caused by weakness may in fact be abnormal hyperactivity of an opposing muscle restricting range of motion and excursion.

Comprehensive retraining incorporates significant education regarding facial anatomy and muscle actions. This is key to comprehending the true nature of the disability, that is, the difference between a deficiency of muscle activity resulting in no movement (flaccidity) and aberrant muscle activity (synkinesis) resulting in wrong movement. In

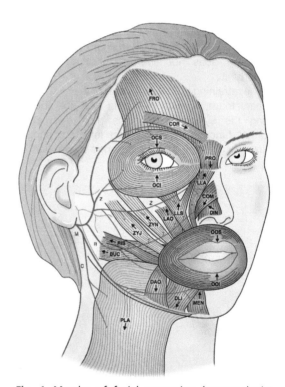

Fig. 1. Muscles of facial expression (arrows depict normal direction of contraction). Muscles: BUC, buccinators; COM, compressor naris; COR, corrugator; DAO, depressor anguli oris; DIN, dilator naris; DLI, depressor labii inferioris; FRO, frontalis; LAO, levator anguli oris; LLA, levator labii alaeque nasi; LLS, levator labii superioris; MEN, mentalis; OCI, orbicularis oculi inferioris; OCS, orbicularis oculi superioris; OOI, orbicularis oris inferioris; OOS, orbicularis oris superioris; PLA, platysma; PRO, procerus; RIS, risorius; ZYJ, zygomaticus major; ZYN, zygomaticus minor. Facial nerve branches: B, buccal; C, cervical; M, mandibular; T, temporal; Z, zygomaticus. (Adapted from Balliet R. Facial paralysis and other neuromuscular dysfunctions of the peripheral nervous system. In: Payton OD. Manual of physical therapy. New York: Churchill Livingstone; 1989. p. 179; with permission.)

cases of synkinesis, the common practice of prescribing maximum effort movements (in an erroneous attempt to strengthen muscles) intensifies the abnormal response, reinforcing the synkinesis. Appropriate intervention focuses on accurately coordinating viable, albeit synkinetic, muscles rather than stimulating flaccid ones. With skilled training it is possible to improve movement patterns and expression even many years after synkinesis develops.[35,36]

When used in conjunction with facial NMR, botulinum toxin provides a "window of opportunity" during which the patient can learn and practice isolated, coordinated movement patterns without the cocontraction and restriction caused by synkinesis. It is preferable to complete 6 months of retraining before injecting botulinum toxin to enable the patient to learn the synkinesis inhibition techniques. The presence of botulinum toxin before retraining does not afford this same learning opportunity.

The retraining therapist, as part of the multidisciplinary team, is instrumental in precisely identifying the synkinetic muscles most restricting normal function. These, when injected, should allow for greater ease and range of motion in

keeping with the patient's stated goals, without causing additional morbidity. Targeting the most appropriate injections sites for the best outcome is challenging owing to the complex interactions of the facial muscles. Knowledge of anatomy is not enough. It is also essential to know the working action of each muscle, both in isolation and in conjunction with the actions of others.

The most common injection sites include the orbicularis oculi, corrugator, platysma, and mentalis muscles (**Fig. 1**). Recently, minimal dose injections to the synkinetic buccinator have proven to be of benefit in improving outcomes.[37] The midfacial muscles are rarely injected to avoid creating weakness in key areas targeted during the NMR process, such as smile. For greatest accuracy in targeting injection sites, the patient is asked to demonstrate the expressions that elicit the synkinetic response. Forceful eye closure, smile, pucker and snarl will most commonly produce the response. Each movement may elicit a unique synkinetic pattern, so all should be tested. It is important to note that even a region demonstrating little to no volitional activity (e.g. forehead) can demonstrate significant aberrant activity in a synkinetic pattern, so should be evaluated in that

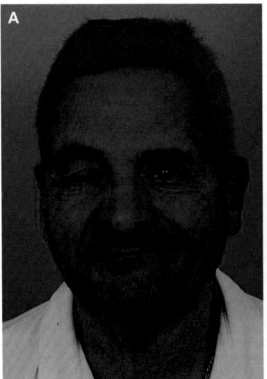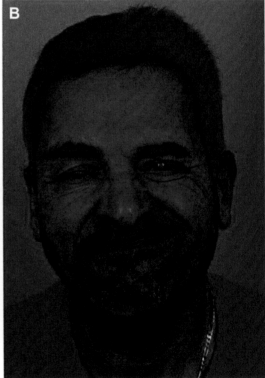

Fig. 2. Treatment of Synkinesis in the Peri-Ocular Area. (*A*) Patient with visible synkinesis in the right orbicularis oculi muscle. Botulinum toxin was injected in the right periorbital area displayed in the figure (doses are in Units, Black = 1cc dilution). (*B*) One month after botulinum treatment showing improved eye opening.

context. (In such a case, no brow movement is observed when the patient attempts to raise it volitionally, however, significant elevation may occur during smile or pucker).

Neuromodulator Injection

When the botulinum toxin vials arrive, they are frozen and need to be reconstituted with normal saline. The authors use 2 main preparations of botulinum toxin, a 1 mL dilution (10 units per each 0.1 mL) and a 2 mL dilution (5 units per each 0.1 mL). The 1 mL dilution provides a solution that allows a more targeted approach to muscle relaxation, particularly in the medial midface zygomatic complex and the periocular areas. The 2 mL dilution allows for much greater diffusion of the toxin, and can be advantageous in larger muscles, such as the platysma.

After the injection, patients should avoid any physical activity or facial exercises for 2 days to prevent diffusion of the product to unwanted areas. Botulinum toxin starts to take effect in 3 to 5 days and the peak effect is routinely seen at 2 weeks. For that reason, we usually recommend that patients follow up 1 month after treatment to assess efficacy of the treatment. At that point, any additional areas that did not respond as well as desired can be treated with additional botulinum toxin. It is highly recommended to begin conservatively with the patient's first treatment, and then titrate the botulinum toxin dose upward as needed.

Periocular

The forehead and periocular area contains the muscles that both elevate and depress the brow complex. The frontalis muscle is the main elevator of the eyebrows, and the corrugator supercilli and orbicularis oculi are the main depressors of the eyebrows. Spasm of the frontalis and corrugator supercilli muscles are frequent causes of tension headache pain in synkinesis patients, and can often be elicited with a careful history and examination. Additionally, one of the most frequent complaints of patients with synkinesis is the tight spasm that can occur in the orbicularis oculi muscle. This causes a narrowing of the visual field in the effected eye, painful spasm of the muscle, and exaggeration of the crow's feet area (Fig. 2).

Midface One of the most challenging areas to inject is the cheek and midface area, because spasm of the zygomatic muscles leads to pain and discomfort in the cheek. Unfortunately, this is the area that is most frequently cited by patients as being the most bothersome in terms of pain and discomfort. The lower face is also the most challenging area to inject. Overinjection of the muscles acting

on the nasolabial fold can result in the lack of function of the smiling muscles and cause great distress to patients for 3 to 4 months until the effect of the drug wears off. Patients most often state that they would prefer the increased muscle tension, rather than looking "paralyzed," with complete muscle inactivity. For this reason, NMR is a critical aspect to address tension in the cheek. Neuromuscular retaining can often be a safer, much more effective intervention than botulinum toxin injection in relieving the painful spasm in the cheek.

Occasionally, one can elicit spasm in the area of the zygomaticus minor muscle, located in the nasolabial fold just about one-third of the distance from the nasal ala to the lateral commissure (**Fig. 3**). A precise injection of botulinum toxin of 0.5 to 1 unit, with a concentrated 1 mL dilution of product to minimize diffusion, can be very effective. Injecting over the malar eminence high and lateral in the cheek is not recommended because this leads frequently to complete weakness of the zygomatic muscle complex.

Perioral The most frequent complaint that we hear from patients is the inability to achieve what

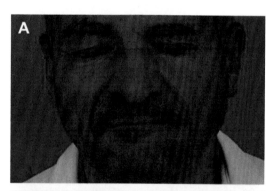
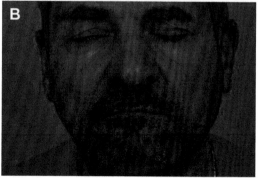

Fig. 3. Spasm of the Zygomaticus Minor. (*A*) In the right hemi-face, forceful eye closure triggers spasm of the right Zygomaticus Minor muscle. Botulinum toxin was injected in the area just anterior to the right nasolabial fold displayed in the figure (doses are in Units, Black = 1cc dilution). (*B*) One month following treatment, there is reduced spasm in the right cheek.

they know as a normal smile. This can be caused by a variety of factors including the downward pull of lip depressor muscles that prevent lateral upward excursion of the lateral commissure. Targeted treatment of the platysma, depressor labi inferioris, and depressore anguli oris is quite helpful. Symmetry of the lower lip, particularly during smiling is very important, and injection of the contralateral lip depressor muscles can often be helpful.

A typically overlooked muscle that can limit lateral excursion of the smile is the buccinator muscle (**Fig. 4**). The Buccinator muscle is an accessory muscle for mastication, but is controlled by the buccal branch of the facial nerve. The muscle's main action is to pull the lateral commissure of the mouth posteriorly and to tense and flatten the mucosal surface of the cheek against the teeth. In doing so, the angle of the mouth is pulled closed. Spasm of the buccinator muscle pulls the corner of the mouth posteriorly on the synkinetic side,

limiting exposure of the upper teeth and upward movement of the smile.

Neck

Tense spasm of the platysma muscle on the affected side is a freqent complaint among synkinesis patients. The medial fibers contribute to the depressor function of the lateral oral commissure, and can act as a pulley that pulls the corner of the mouth in a downward direction. This downward traction of the platysma muscle interferes with smiling as it acts against the zygomatic muscles to allow upward and lateral excursion of the oral commissure. As a result, after treating the platysma muscle with botulinum toxin, patients usually report improvement in their ability to smile on the affected side. Typical injection doses in the platysma muscle are 15 to 20 U of botulinum toxin (**Fig. 6**). We typically use 2 cc dilutions to facilitate even spread of the drug within the muscle.

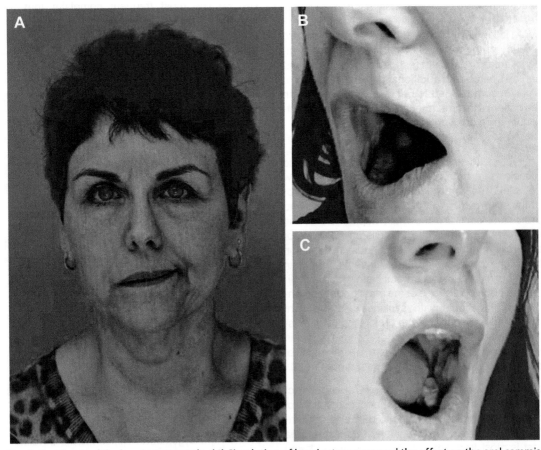

Fig. 4. Synkinesis of the buccinator muscle. (*A*) Simulation of buccinator spasm and the effect on the oral commissure. This patient had left facial synkinesis, with image (*B*) displaying the normal, unaffected side. Compare to (*C*), showing synkinetic muscular activity upon forcefull eye closure. Note the spasm and bulge of the buccinator muscle.

Contralateral Normal Side: Addressing Asymmetries

In many patients, the perception of asymmetry can be the most troubling to them, and can be very bothersome during normal conversation. The 2 most common offenders are the periocular and lateral commissure. Overactivity in these areas during laughing or conveying emotions can amplify and draw attention to the patient's facial asymmetry. Both young and old patients are affected, but age related changes amplify this effect.

When addressing the synkinetic hemiface with botulinum injections, the contralateral normal corrugator and orbicularis oculi are also addressed. This can reduce the appearance of an unsightly bulge of the corrugator muscle and crow's feet on the normal side. It is also very important to consider the position of the patient's eyebrows on the normal side. Increased resting tone of the depressor muscles on the affected synkinetic side can cause the eyebrow to be positioned lower. Therefore, the eyebrows can be evened out by placing a relatively lower dose of botulinum toxin on the normal side, and a higher dose on the synkinetic spastic side. The same concept can be applied where increased resting tone of the frontalis causes the eyebrow to be higher on the affected synkinetic side.

Abnormalities of the smile can be one of the most frequent complaints in patients with synkinesis. Patients with a full denture smile, as described by Rubin,[37,38] can be particularly susceptible. Overpull of the zygomatic muscles that elevate the lateral commissure, and the depressor anguli oris and depressor labii inferioris that depress the lip, can greatly exaggerate the asymmetries during smiling or laughing. Injecting botulinum toxin in the zygomatic elevator muscles is a slippery slope, and must be done with great trepidation. Dosing is typically done with 0.5 to 1 unit just lateral to the oral commissure.

Botulinum injection in the contralateral lip depressor muscles can help produce a dramatic improvement in the symmetry of the smile (**Fig. 5**). It is important, however, to diagnose whether the overactive downward pull is owing to the depressor labii inferioris, depressor anguli oris, or both. The depressor anguli oris is a broader muscle that typically requires a greater dosage (3–5 U) than its more medial counterpart depressor labii inferioris (1–3 U).

Risks

Botulinum toxin treatment is very well-tolerated and has minimal risks to the patient. Care should be taken, however, because facial paralysis

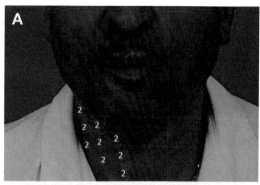

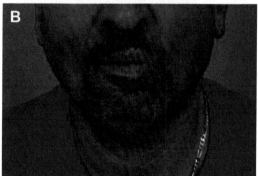

Fig. 5. Platysma Muscle Synkinesis. Treatment of Synkinesis in the Peri-Ocular Area. (*A*) Patient with visible synkinesis in the right Platysma muscle triggered by lip puckering. Botulinum toxin was injected into neck displayed in the figure (doses are in Units, Yellow = 2cc dilution). (*B*) One month after botulinum treatment showing improved eye opening.

patients typically require a higher dose than the common cosmetic patient. Some of the more common risks include slight bruising after injections.

ALTERNATIVE TREATMENTS

Treatment of synkinesis with botulinum toxin is relatively easy, requires no downtime for the patient, and is quite reproducible. For this reason, botulinum toxin injection has become the standard of care for patients with synkinesis. Neurolysis has experienced a return to practice, and this procedure was historically once the main treatment for synkinesis. Selective mymectomy has been an alternative treatment for a more permanent relief of synkinesis. Mymectomy has been offered for many of the facial muscles, but may be the most effective for overcontraction of the stapedius muscle, causing a loud irritating noise from movement of the tympanic membrane with facial movement. The most common mymectomy performed today, however, is transection of the platysma muscle (**Fig. 6**), performed through a 2-cm incision in a neck crease. A history of relief of pain and discomfort from synkinesis with botulinum toxin injections is usually a good predictor of a successful mymectomy.

FUTURE DIRECTIONS

One of the downsides of neuromodulator treatment of synkinesis is that injections must be repeated every 3 months. Second, injections are performed with very small needles and are quite well-tolerated; however, there is some discomfort associated with the treatment. One new pharmaceutical company, Revance Therapeutics, has developed new neuromodulators to address some of these issues.

The first product, RT001, is a topical gel formulation of the botulinum toxin type 1.[39] The drug is applied to the skin at precise locations, and after sufficient time is absorbed and delivers its effect. The company is targeting a cosmetic indication for crow's feet lines. The drug has shown promising results in more than 17 clinical studies and is currently in phase III clinical trials. Topical RT001 has not been studied in synkinesis, but it seems ideally positioned to address synkinetic facial muscles that located more superficially in the facial soft tissues, such as the orbicularis oculi and orbicularis oris. A superficial location and nearby proximity to the skin would theoretically minimize the distance for absorption and have a greater chance of success.

The second product, RT002, is a new injectable formulation of the botulinum toxin that was designed to offer a more target delivery of the botulinum toxin and reduce the spread of toxin beyond the site of injection.[40] Again, RT002 has not been studied in synkinesis patients, but seems ideally suited to precisely target a facial muscle in spasm, while sparing a nearby, uninvolved muscle. RT002 has currently completed phase II clinical trials for cosmetic glabellar frown lines and functional cervical dystonia. One encouraging finding from the clinical studies was that RT002 achieved a median duration effect of 7 months. The longer duration of effect might reduce the number of visits that synkinesis patients typically need.

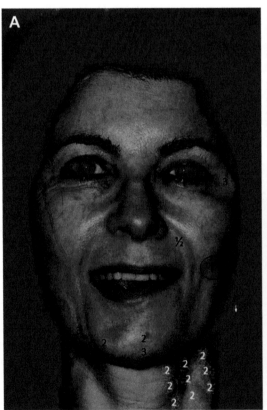 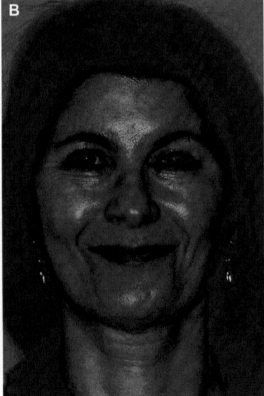

Fig. 6. Injection of contralateral lip depressors improves the smile. (*A*) Patient with visible synkinesis in the left hemiface, botulinum toxin was injected into the affected left face, and the contralateral right lip depressors (doses are in Units, Black = 1cc dilution; Yellow = 2cc dilution). (*B*) One month after botulinum treatment showing a balanced smile.

REFERENCES

1. Guerrissi JO. Selective myectomy for postparetic facial synkinesis. Plast Reconstr Surg 1991;87: 459–66.
2. Chen C-K, Tang Y-B. Myectomy and botulinum toxin for paralysis of the marginal mandibular branch of the facial nerve: a series of 76 cases. Plast Reconstr Surg 2007;120(7):1859–64.
3. Terzis JK, Karypidis D. Therapeutic strategies in post-facial paralysis synkinesis in pediatric patients. J Plast Reconstr Aesthet Surg 2012;65(8): 1009–18.
4. Chuang DC, Chang TN, Lu JC. Postparalysis facial sykinesis: clinical classification and surgical strategies. Plast Reconstr Surg Glob Open 2015; 3:e320.
5. Haykal S, Arad E, Bagher S, et al. The role of Botulinum Toxin A in the establishment of symmetry in pediatric analysis of the lower lip. JAMA Facial Plast Surg 2015;17(3):174–8.
6. Azuma T, Nakamura K, Takahashi M, et al. Mirror biofeedback rehabilitation after administration of single-dose botulinum toxin for treatment of facial synkinesis. Otolaryngol Head Neck Surg 2012;146: 40–5.
7. Lee JM, Choi KH, Lim BW, et al. Half-mirror biofeedback exercise in combination with three botulinum toxin A injections for long-lasting treatment of facial sequelae after facial paralysis. J Plast Reconstr Aesthet Surg 2015; 68(1):71–8.
8. Chen JJ, Dashtipour K. Abo-, inco-, ona-, and rima-botulinum toxins in clinical therapy: a primer. Pharmacotherapy 2013;33(3):304–18.
9. Toffola ED, Furini F, Redaelli C, et al. Evaluation and treatment of synkinesis with botulinum toxin following facial nerve palsy. Disabil Rehabil 2010; 32(17):1414–8.
10. Armstrong MW, Mountain RE, Murray JA. Treatment of facial synkinesis and facial asymmetry with botulinum toxin type A following facial nerve palsy. Clin Otolaryngol Allied Sci 1996;21(1):15–20.
11. Couch SM, Chundury RV, Holds JB. Subjective and objective outcome measures in the treatment of facial nerve synkinesis with onabotulinumtoxinA (Botox). Ophthal Plast Reconstr Surg 2014;30(3): 246–50.
12. Borodic GE, Pearce LB, Cheney M, et al. Botulinum A toxin for treatment of aberrant facial nerve regeneration. Plast Reconstr Surg 1993;91:1042–5.
13. Scott AB. Botulinum toxin injection into extraocular muscles as an alternative to strabismus surgery. Ophthalmology 1980;87:1044–9.
14. Carruthers JD, Carruthers JA. Treatment of glabellar frown lines with C. Botulinum A exotoxin. J Dermatol Surg Oncol 1992;18:17–21.
15. Borodic G, Bartley M, Slattery W, et al. Botulinum toxin for aberrant facial nerve regeneration: double-blind, placebo controlled trial using subjective endpoints. Plast Reconstr Surg 2005;116(1):36–43.
16. Mehta RP, Hadlock T. Botulinum toxin and quality of life in patients with facial paralysis. Arch Facial Plast Surg 2014;10(2):84–7.
17. Ross BG, Fradet G, Nedzelski JM. Development of a sensitive clinical facial grading system. Eur Arch Otorhinolaryngol 1994;S180–1.
18. Mehta RP, WernickRobinson M, Hadlock TA. Validation of the synkinesis assessment questionnaire. Laryngoscope 2007;117(5):923–6.
19. Filipo R, Spahiu I, Covelli E, et al. Botulinum toxin in the treatment of facial synkinesis and hyperkinesis. Laryngoscope 2012;122:266–70.
20. Putterman AM. Botulinum toxin injections in the treatment of seventh nerve misdirection. Am J Ophthalmol 1990;110:205–6.
21. Chua CN, Quhill F, Jones E, et al. Treatment of aberrant facial nerve regeneration with botulinum toxin A. Orbit 2004;23(4):213–8.
22. Rogers CR, Schmidt KL, VanSwearingen JM, et al. Automated facial image analysis: detecting improvement in abnormal facial movement after treatment with botulinum toxin A. Ann Plast Surg 2007;58(1):39–47.
23. de Maio M, Bento RF. Botulinum toxin in facial palsy: an effective treatment for contralateral hyperkinesis. Plast Reconstr Surg 2007;120(4):917–27.
24. Salles AG, Toledo PN, Ferreira MC. Botulinum toxin injection in long standing facial paralysis patients: improvement of facial symmetry observed up to 6 months. Aesthetic Plast Surg 2009;33(4):582–90.
25. Kollewe K, Mohammadi B, Dengler R, et al. Hemifacial spasm and reinnervation synkinesias: long-term treatment with either Botox or Dysport. J Neural Transm 2010;117(6):759–63.
26. Monini S, De Carlo A, Biagini M, et al. Combined protocol for treatment of secondary effects from facial nerve palsy. Acta Otolaryngol 2011;131(8): 882–6.
27. Sadiq S, Khwaja S, Saeed S. Botulinum toxin to improve lower facial symmetry in facial nerve palsy. Eye 2012;73(11):1431–6.
28. McElhinny ER, Reich I, Burt B, et al. Treatment of pseudoptosis secondary to aberrant regeneration of the facial nerve with botulinum toxin type A. Ophthal Plast Reconstr Surg 2013;29(3):175–8.
29. Choi KH, Rho SH, Lee JM, et al. Botulinum toxin injection of both sides of the face to treat post-paralytic facial synkinesis. J Plast Reconstr Aesthet Surg 2013;66(8):1058–63.
30. Montserrat L, Benito M, Jankovic J, et al. Facial synkinesis and aberrant regeneration of facial nerve. In: Advances in neurology: facial dyskinesias, vol. 49. New York Raven Press; 1988. p. 211–24.

31. Bacsi AM, Kiernan MC. Changes in axonal excitability and burst pattern behaviour in synkinesis. J Clin Neurosci 2008;15(11):1288–90.

32. Maeyama H, Aoyagi M, Tojima H, et al. Electrophysiological study on the pathology of synkinesis after facial nerve paralysis. Acta Otolaryngol Suppl 1994;511:161–4.

33. Moran CJ, Neely JG. Patterns of facial nerve synkinesis. Laryngoscope 1996;106(12):1491–6.

34. Basmajian JV, DeLuca CJ. Muscles Alive: Their Functions Revealed by Electromyography. Baltimore: Williams & Wilkins; 1985.

35. Diels HJ, Beurskens C. Neuromuscular Retraining: Non-Surgical Therapy for Facial Palsy. In: Slattery W, Azizzadeh B, editors. The Facial Nerve. New York: Thieme; 2014. p. 205–12.

36. Balliet R, Shinn JB, Bach-y-Rita P. Facial paralysis rehabilitation: retraining selective muscle control. Int Rehabil Med 1982;4(2):67–74.

37. Wei L, Diels J, Lucarelli M. Treating buccinator with botulinum toxin in patients with facial synkinesis - a previously overlooked target. Ophthal Plast Reconstr Surg 2015. [Epub ahead of print].

38. Rubin LR. The anatomy of a smile: its importance in the treatment of facial paralysis. Plast Reconstr Surg 1974;53:384–7.

39. Brandt F, O'Connell C, Cazzaniga A, et al. Efficacy and safety evaluation of a novel botulinum toxin topical gel for the treatment of moderate to severe lateral canthal lines. Derm Surg 2010;36(S4):2111–8.

40. Stone HF, Zhu Z, Thach T, et al. Characterization of diffusion and duration of action of a new botulinum toxin type A formulation. Toxicon 2011;58:159–67.

Management of the Eye in Facial Paralysis

John J. Chi, MD

KEYWORDS

- Facial paralysis • Facial palsy • Lagophthalmos • Ectropion • Upper eyelid weight
- Upper eyelid loading • Lower eyelid tightening • Eyelid reanimation

KEY POINTS

- Upper eyelid loading procedures are the gold standard for surgical management of lagophthalmos in the setting of a paralyzed upper eyelid.
- Lower eyelid tightening procedures reposition the lower eyelid and help to maintain the aqueous tear film of the eye.
- Lagophthalmos secondary to facial paralysis causes poor tear film movement and tear evaporation, which can lead to exposure keratitis, corneal abrasion, and permanent vision changes.
- Eyelid reanimation restores the protective functions vital to ocular preservation, which is particularly important because these patients often have multiple nervous deficits, including corneal anesthesia.
- Nonoperative management of patients with eyelid paralysis should be reserved for patients with reliable access to regular ophthalmologic examinations, overall good health, and minimal comorbidities.

INTRODUCTION

Facial paralysis has many devastating psychological, social, and physiologic consequences. Of the physiologic concerns, ocular preservation is the first and foremost priority in the management of the patient with facial paralysis. Medical and surgical interventions should be used as appropriate to ensure ocular safety and health. Appropriate patient education regarding the dangers of exposure keratitis is an important aspect of patient care. The management of the eye in facial paralysis may be led by the facial plastic surgeon, plastic surgeon, oculoplastic surgeon, or otolaryngologist, but early and effective communication and coordination of care between the patient, the ophthalmologist, and the surgeon managing the patient with facial paralysis is critical.

Upper eyelid loading for the treatment of paralytic lagophthalmos was first described in 1950 by Sheehan[1] and popularized by Jobe[2] in 1974. Lid loading procedures rely on gravitational forces to close the paralyzed upper eyelid by overcoming the action of the levator palpebrae superioris. Lower eyelid tightening is often implemented in conjunction with upper eyelid loading. As with all reanimation procedures in the paralyzed face, lid loading and lower eyelid tightening serve to restore the form and function of the paralyzed face.[3–5] Eyelid reanimation can restore a static and dynamic symmetry to the eyes, but more importantly restores the protective functions that are vital to ocular preservation. These considerations are particularly important because these patients often have multiple cranial nerve deficits, such as corneal anesthesia and extraocular muscle paralysis. Other procedures for the paralyzed eyelids include tarsorrhaphy, spring implantation, and temporalis muscle transposition. However,

Disclosure Statement: The author has no conflicts of interest or financial disclosures to disclose.
Division of Facial Plastic & Reconstructive Surgery, Washington University Facial Plastic Surgery Center, Washington University in St Louis–School of Medicine, 1020 North Mason Road, Medical Building 3, Suite 205, St Louis, MO 63141, USA
E-mail address: JChi@wustl.edu

Facial Plast Surg Clin N Am 24 (2016) 21–28
http://dx.doi.org/10.1016/j.fsc.2015.09.003
1064-7406/16/$ – see front matter © 2016 Elsevier Inc. All rights reserved.

their associated side effects and complications have left them with little, if any, indications for use today.

ASSESSMENT OF THE EYE IN FACIAL PARALYSIS

The preoperative assessment of the facial paralysis patient is a critical component of their surgical management. The etiology and severity of the facial nerve paralysis must be accurately assessed before intervention.[4,5] A detailed history of ocular issues before and since the onset of facial paralysis is an important part of the initial assessment. Pre-existing ocular conditions, such as prior ophthalmologic surgery, chronic lid infections, ptosis, or refractive errors, may be exacerbated by the facial paralysis. Additionally, any and all prior interventions to manage the paralyzed eyelids must be documented. If the affected eye is the only seeing eye or the better seeing eye, then extra precautions must be taken ensure its health and safety. The physical examination of the patient with facial paralysis should include visual acuity, extraocular muscle assessment, visual fields, lacrimal secretion, corneal sensation, pupillary assessment, lower eyelid position, margin gap, and the presence or absence of a Bell's phenomenon. Assessment of the marginal reflex distances 1 (MRD1) and 2 (MRD2) is also useful in assessing for ptosis and ectropion. The MRD1 is the distance from the pupillary light reflex to the upper eyelid. The MRD2 is the distance from the pupillary light reflex to the lower eyelid. The margin gap is the distance between the margin of the upper and lower eyelid with involuntary blink and maximal effort. The palpebral fissure height is the distance between the upper and lower eyelid in primary gaze. All patients with facial paralysis should be evaluated by an ophthalmologist to perform a baseline ophthalmologic examination and to establish care with an ophthalmologist (**Tables 1** and **2**).

Patients may present with good eye closure, but a poor blink response. These patients remain at risk for keratitis, owing to a loss of the windshield wiper effect of the blink with subsequent poor wetting of the cornea. Other patients may present with good eye closure while upright, but poor eye closure when supine. Although these patients seem to have good eye closure, consideration should be made for supplemental ocular lubrication, moisture chamber, or nighttime taping, if not surgical intervention. The presence or absence of a Bell's phenomenon should also be noted. These patients are better able to tolerate poor eye closure because the cornea is protected underneath the upper eyelid with a brisk

Table 1
History and physical examination of the eye in facial paralysis

History	Physical Examination
Comprehensive medical history	Comprehensive physical examination
Premorbid ocular symptoms	Eyebrow position
New ocular symptoms	Upper and lower eyelid position
Prior ophthalmologic surgery	Extraocular muscle movements
Prior facial reanimation surgery	Margin gap with blink and maximal effort
	Marginal reflex distance (MRD); MRD1, MRD2
	Palpebral fissure height
	Corneal sensation
	Pupillary assessment
	Bell's phenomenon
	Fundoscopy

Bell's phenomenon. Acute postoperative lateral skull base surgery patients with a complete facial paralysis may initially present with almost normal appearing eye closure, presumably owing to edema of the eyelids and orbicularis oculi muscle. However, lagophthalmos eventually develops after this immediate postoperative period. Corneal sensation should be assessed and compared with the unaffected side. Lacrimal secretion can be assessed using Schirmer's test. Although eyelid approximation depends primarily on the movement of the upper eyelid, the position and slight movement of the lower eyelid is also important in ocular protection. Deviation of the lower eyelid from its normal position at the lower limbus owing to paralytic ectropion can impact the maintenance of an appropriate

Table 2
Testing of the eye in facial paralysis

Test	Purpose
Visual acuity	Baseline visual acuity
Slit-lamp examination	Assess cornea, eyelids, conjunctiva, sclera, iris
Schirmer's test	Assess aqueous tear production
Jones test	Assessment of physiologic nasolacrimal drainage
Visual fields	Visual field limitations

tear film causing dryness or epiphora, and even diminish the benefits of supplemental lubrication. In the setting of lower eyelid malposition, lower eyelid repositioning or tightening procedures should be considered to ensure adequate corneal protection.[3] Lagophthalmos and ectropion secondary to facial paralysis cause poor tear film movement and tear evaporation, which can lead to exposure keratitis, corneal abrasion, and permanent vision changes, including blindness.[4–6]

INDICATIONS FOR SURGICAL INTERVENTION

The etiology and severity of the facial paralysis is an important factor in the management of the paralyzed eyelids. Upper eyelid loading procedures are usually indicated for patients with incomplete eye closure in whom spontaneous recovery is expected to be prolonged and/or incomplete. Additional indications include patients with a poor Bell's phenomenon or sequelae of corneal exposure. Patients demonstrating rapid improvement of a facial paralysis may be considered for management with supplemental lubrication, moisture chambers, nighttime taping, and possibly a temporary tarsorrhaphy for a period of time to see if the eyelid function returns. Medical management for patients with upper eyelid paralysis should be reserved for patients with reliable access to regular ophthalmologic examinations, overall good health, and minimal other comorbidities. Upper eyelid loading procedures are the gold standard for surgical management of lagophthalmos in the setting of a paralyzed upper eyelid. These procedures are reversible and generally performed under local anesthesia.

Preoperative testing in the office to determine the appropriate size weight is an important step in surgical planning (**Fig. 1**). The test weight is centered over the medial limbus and is secured with double-sided adhesive to the upper eyelid. The weight is left attached for several minutes. The appropriate size weight allows effective eye closure without inducing ptosis. Eye closure should be assessed with the patient in the upright and supine positions to approximate the position of the weight and globe when the patient is awake and sleeping. Most patients require a 0.8, 1.0 or 1.2 g weight.

Lower eyelid tightening procedures are indicated for patients with paralytic ectropion who have pooling of tears, epiphora, eversion of the lacrimal punctum, a disfiguring lower eyelid position (MRD2 of >5 mm or significantly different from the nonparalyzed eye) or a significant margin gap.

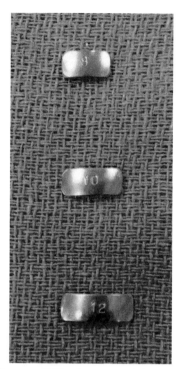

Fig. 1. Upper eyelid implant test weights: 0.8, 1.0, and 1.2 g.

RELEVANT ANATOMY

The skin and subcutaneous tissue of the upper eyelid are very thin and pliable. The supratarsal crease is created by the attachments of the levator aponeurosis directly into the eyelid skin. It is usually located 6 to 10 mm above the lash line in the midpupillary line. The orbicularis oculi muscle covers the upper eyelid and is found deep to the skin and subcutaneous tissue (**Fig. 2**). Superiorly on the upper eyelid, the orbital septum and superior attachments of the levator aponeurosis to the tarsal plate are deep to the orbicularis oculi. Inferiorly on the upper eyelid, the anterior attachments of the levator aponeurosis to the tarsal plate and the tarsal plate are deep to the orbicularis oculi. Deep to the tarsal plate is the conjunctiva. The levator palpebrae superioris and Müller's muscles are upper eyelid retractors. Preservation of their muscular attachments to the tarsal plate is critical to the prevention of postoperative ptosis. Despite good surgical technique, postoperative ptosis may occur. This phenomenon may be transient and resolve over several weeks with accommodation by the upper eyelid retractors. If the ptosis persists, then it may be necessary to replace the upper eyelid implant with a smaller weight. This possibility should be discussed with the patient preoperatively.

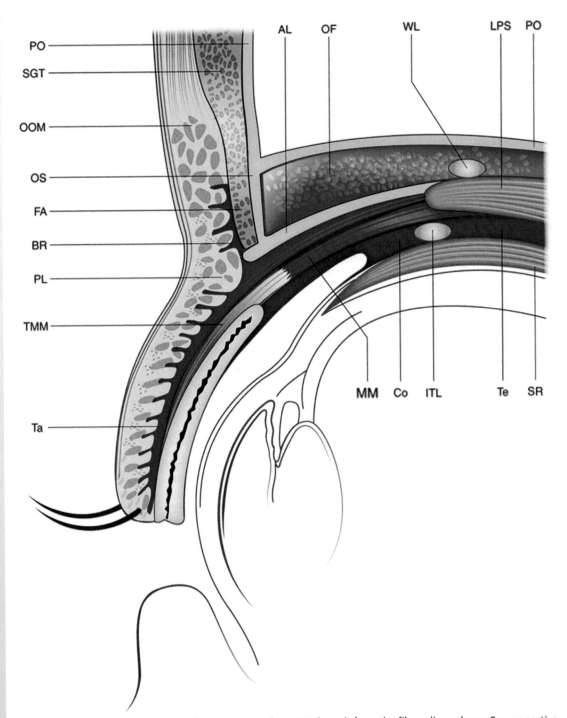

Fig. 2. Cross-section of the upper eyelid. AL, anterior layer; BR, branch from the fibroadipose layer; Co, connective tissue; FA, fibroadipose layer; ITL, intermuscular transverse ligament; LPS, levator palpebrae superioris muscle; MM, Müller's muscle; OF, orbital fat; OOM, orbicularis oculi muscle; OS, orbital septum; PL, posterior layer; PO, periorbita; SGT, subgaleal tissue; SR, superior rectus muscle; Ta, tarsus; Te, Tenon capsule; TMM, tendon of Müller muscle; WL, Whitnall ligament. (*From* Lam VB, Czyz CN, Wulc AE. The brow-lid continuum: an anatomic perspective. Clin Plast Surg 2013;40:8; with permission.)

The lower eyelid anatomy is similar to that of the upper eyelid; the skin and subcutaneous tissues are very thin and pliable. The lower eyelid is divided into 3 layers. The anterior lamella is composed of the skin and orbicularis oculi muscle. The middle lamella is composed of the orbital septum. The posterior lamella is composed of the tarsal plate and conjunctiva.

OPERATIVE TECHNIQUE: UPPER EYELID LOADING

Insertion of an upper eyelid weight involves a horizontal skin incision, dissection to the tarsal plate, creation of a pocket between the orbicularis oculi and the tarsal plate, and fixation of the implant to the tarsal plate. Although other locations for implant placement have been described (ie, septal, orbital), pretarsal implant placement is the technique most commonly used by practicing facial plastic surgeons, ophthalmologists, otolaryngologists, and plastic surgeons.[2,6] Therefore, the discussion herein focuses on this technique.

Upper eyelid loading procedures are usually performed under local anesthesia in an office or operating room setting. Patients that are unable to tolerate this procedure under local anesthesia may try a mild oral sedative in conjunction with a local anesthetic before planning for a procedure under general anesthesia. Preoperative testing is performed to determine the appropriate size weight.

After comfortably positioning the patient, the incision is marked. The incision is centered at the medial limbus and located approximately 6 to 8 mm superior to the lid margin, either at or just inferior to the supratarsal crease. Topical anesthesia is then applied to the cornea. Next, approximately 0.5 mL of 1% lidocaine with 1:100,000 epinephrine is injected into the incision. Balancing appropriate anesthesia with tissue distortion from infiltration is an important consideration. The surgical field is then prepped with skin preparation solution taking care not to expose the cornea to this agent. A corneal protector is then placed over the eye.

A no. 15 blade scalpel is used to incise the skin. The subcutaneous dissection and division of the orbicularis oculi can be performed sharply with a scalpel or scissors. Hemostasis can be achieved using electrocautery or thermal cautery. If thermal cautery is implemented, appropriate fire safety precautions should be taken. Dissection is then carried through the orbicularis oculi down to the tarsal plate. Special attention should be paid to avoid transecting the superior attachments of the levator aponeurosis and Müller's muscle to the tarsal plate.

Once the dissection is on the tarsal plate, a pocket for implant placement should be dissected with curved, sharp scissors. The pocket should be the approximate width of the implant extending down to the lid margin. Ideally, the implant should be centered over the medial limbus and placed inferiorly at the lid margin. Dissection superiorly along the tarsal plate should be kept at a minimum to avoid transecting the attachments of the levator aponeurosis and Müller's muscle to the tarsal plate.

The implant is then secured to the tarsal plate using a 6-0 clear monofilament, nonabsorbable suture passed through the perforations in the implant and passed partial thickness through the tarsal plate. The implant should be seated flush against the tarsal plate without buckling the native contour of the tarsal plate. The orbicularis oculi is closed using 5-0 undyed monofilament, absorbable suture. The skin is closed using 6-0 fast-absorbing suture or 6-0 dyed monofilament, nonabsorbable suture, depending on the surgeon's preference. Small bites of tissue should be taken when closing the orbicularis oculi and skin to avoid vertical lid shortening.

Postoperative care includes a topical ophthalmic antibiotic ointment applied for 5 days. Oral antibiotics are generally not indicated.

PEARLS: UPPER EYELID LOADING

Complications of upper eyelid loading procedures include extrusion, migration, poor aesthetics (visible scar, implant visible owing to thin skin, implant visible owing to contour irregularity), ptosis, and vertical lid shortening. Modifications to the implant have been developed to mitigate some of these complications. Platinum implants are more dense than gold allowing a significantly thinner profile. Platinum chain implants have the additional advantage of superior contour match with the upper eyelid tarsus.

Avoid Upper Eyelid Ptosis

Place the skin incision over the tarsal plate. Incisions located too far superiorly can lead to unnecessary dissection inferiorly to reach the tarsal plate and risk division of the levator aponeurosis and Müller's muscle attachments to the tarsal plate, which can lead to ptosis of the upper eyelid. In patients where the supratarsal crease is located far above the superior extent of the tarsal plate, this complication becomes more of a concern.

Avoid Upper Eyelid Vertical Lid Shortening

During wound closure, take small bites of the orbicularis oculi and upper eyelid skin to minimize the possibility of vertical lid shortening. This wound is usually not under tension and does not require significant tissue overlap to ensure closure.

Avoid Implant Visibility

Preserve the superficial tissues overlying the tarsal plate. Thinning of this tissue during dissection can increase implant visibility through the skin. During the suturing of the implant to the tarsal plate, take care to avoid buckling the tarsal plate. The implant should be secured in place without deforming the underlying tarsal plate to ensure that the implant is seated as flush as possible against the tarsal plate.

Use the Existing Fibrous Capsule in Revision Procedures

In the setting of revision upper eyelid loading for extrusion, malposition, or improper weight, remove the existing weight and if at all possible dissect a new pocket deep to its investing fibrous capsule. In this way, the deep aspect of its fibrous capsule can be used as an additional investing layer superficial to the new implant.

MODIFIED UPPER EYELID APPROACHES

Various upper eyelid approaches have also been developed to minimize complications.[6] The traditional approach uses a skin incision at or just inferior to the supratarsal crease and dissection down to the tarsal plate with pretarsal implant placement. This technique is described in the Operative Technique section. This approach divides many of the anterior attachments of the levator aponeurosis to the tarsal plate and risks division of the superior attachments as well. Furthermore, appropriate inferior placement of the implant requires judicious dissection inferiorly to the lid margin. The scar is well-concealed in the supratarsal crease.

A retrograde approach places the skin incision and dissection down to the tarsal plate at the lid margin (~2 mm superior to the lash line). The implant pocket is then dissected superiorly between the tarsal plate and orbicularis oculi muscle. This approach preserves more of the anterior attachments of the levator aponeurosis and does not risk division of the superior attachments. Additionally, the lid margin incision allows the weight to be placed more precisely in an inferior position on the tarsal plate, increasing its efficacy in closing the eye. However, the scar is more visible and in theory the implant is at greater risk for extrusion owing to the inferior position of the incision.

The modified retrograde approach combines the theoretic advantages of the two aforementioned approaches. Like the traditional approach, it uses the supratarsal crease for skin incision. In contrast with the traditional approach, the inferior dissection occurs in the plane between the skin and orbicularis oculi muscle. Like the retrograde approach, the transition through the orbicularis oculi muscle to the tarsal plate occurs at the lid margin and then the implant pocket is dissected superiorly between the tarsal plate and orbicularis oculi muscle. The potential benefits of this approach are that the scar is well-concealed, the implant is more easily positioned inferiorly on the tarsal plate and the attachments of the levator aponeurosis are preserved. However, the implementation of this approach can be difficult because the plane between the skin and orbicularis oculi muscle is not easily traversed.

Septal implant placement uses an upper eyelid incision with dissection through the orbicularis oculi down to the orbital septum and superior tarsal plate. The implant is then secured to the septum and superior tarsal plate.

Orbital implant placement uses the same approach as septal implant placement, however, the orbital septum is divided and the implant is placed postseptal within the orbit. Both of these approaches have the potential for scarring of the orbital septum with accompanying tethering and vertical lid shortening. Additionally, the development of astigmatism is more of a concern with these approaches.[6]

OPERATIVE TECHNIQUE: LOWER EYELID TIGHTENING

Lower eyelid tightening can be performed from a lateral or a medial approach. Laterally based tightening is the surgical technique most commonly performed and, therefore, the discussion herein focuses on this technique; however, medial approaches to lower eyelid tightening are increasing in popularity among oculoplastic surgeons.

Lower eyelid tightening procedures may be performed under local anesthesia in an office or operating room setting. Patients unable to tolerate this procedure under local anesthesia may try a mild oral sedative in conjunction with a local anesthetic before planning for a procedure under general anesthesia.

After comfortably positioning the patient, the incision is marked. The incision is placed at the lateral canthus extending laterally for approximately 1 cm. Topical anesthesia is then applied to the cornea. Next, approximately 0.5 mL of 1% lidocaine with 1:100,000 epinephrine is injected into the incision. Balancing appropriate anesthesia with tissue distortion from infiltration is an important consideration. The surgical field is then prepped with skin preparation solution taking care not to expose the cornea to this agent. A corneal protector is then placed over the eye.

A no. 15 blade scalpel is used to incise the skin. The subcutaneous dissection and division of the orbicularis oculi can be performed sharply with a scalpel or scissors. Hemostasis can be achieved using electrocautery or thermal cautery. If thermal cautery is implemented, appropriate fire safety precautions should be taken. Needle tip electrocautery should then be used to score the lateral orbital rim at the position of the attachment of the lateral canthus to the lateral orbital rim. This point will then serve as a guide for the location of the resuspension of the lateral canthus. Next, using scissors perform the canthotomy and cantholysis. After this step, there should be a significant increase in the laxity of the lower eyelid and it should freely swing inferiorly. When handling the lower eyelid, be careful not to crush the eyelid margin because an injury can cause a postoperative notch at the eyelid margin. Using a fine scissors, strip the mucosa and epithelium from the lateral aspect of the lateral canthal tendon. Be sure to remove all of the meibomian gland tissue. Because the lateral canthal tendon is being advanced into the orbit, a small triangle of redundant skin inferior and lateral to the lateral canthus may need to be excised. Advance the lateral canthus into the medial aspect of the lateral orbital rim at the scoring mark identifying the site of the previous lateral canthal attachment with the appropriate amount of tension to adequately reposition the lower eyelid without causing proptosis, worsening scleral show, or inversion of the lower eyelid lash line. Lateral canthal resuspension is performed with a double-armed 4-0 braided, absorbable polyglycolic acid suture. The needle size should be sufficiently small for ophthalmologic surgery. Pass both needles of this suture through the stripped portion of the lateral canthus. The needles should be passed vertical to one another from the medial aspect of the canthal tendon toward the lateral aspect. The needles should again be passed from the medial aspect of the orbit and away from the globe through the periosteum of the medial surface of the lateral orbital rim. These passes should be made at the scoring mark identifying the previous attachment of the lateral canthal tendon. Do not tie this suture until after the lateral canthus is reconstructed. This ensures that the lateral canthal resuspension does not distort the lateral canthal angle or create too much tension along the

lower eyelid. The lateral canthal reconstruction should recreate the acute angle of the lateral canthus. Using a 6-0 fast-absorbing suture, reapproximate the gray line of the upper and lower eyelid at the lateral canthus with an interrupted suture through the gray lines and the eyelid skin. Next, pass a horizontal mattress suture medial to this knot. Leaving this knot with a long tail, then run the skin closure laterally over the long tail of the knot to secure it away from the cornea and conjunctiva. The deeper tissues of the lateral orbital rim should be closed with a 5-0 braided, absorbable polyglycolic acid suture.

Graft material, such as an acellular dermal matrix, conchal cartilage, or palatal mucosa, may be used for additional lower eyelid structural support. Great care should be taken to bury knots and sutures when securing this graft material so as not to cause postoperative irritation of the cornea and conjunctiva. Some authors also suggest using a midfacial lift in conjunction with a lower eyelid tightening procedure.[7]

Postoperative care includes a topical ophthalmic antibiotic ointment applied for 5 days. Oral antibiotics are generally not indicated.

PEARLS: LOWER EYELID TIGHTENING

Complications of lower eyelid tightening procedures include blunting of the lateral canthal angle, malposition of the lateral canthus, persistent ectropion, entropion, hypertrophic scarring, and poor aesthetics.

Avoid Blunting (Fish Mouth) at the Lateral Canthal Angle

Reapproximate the grayline of the upper and lower eyelid with a horizontal mattress suture to create a sharp angle at the lateral canthus.

Avoid Malposition of the Lateral Canthus

During the dissection onto the lateral orbital rim, score the approximate location of the lateral canthal tendon attachment to the lateral orbital rim. This mark will then serve as a guide for the location of the resuspension of the lateral canthus.

Avoid Overtightening the Lower Eyelid

Before resuspension, assess the position of the globe and lash line relative to the lower eyelid tension created by the resuspension of the lateral canthus. Be sure not to create proptosis, worsening scleral show, or inversion of the lower eyelid lash line by overtightening.

Avoid Postoperative Corneal Abrasions

Any sutures that are left outside the skin should be tied with a long tail. The long tail should then be secured sufficiently away from the cornea either with another knot or adhesive to prevent suture-related trauma to the cornea.

SUMMARY

Ocular preservation is the first and foremost priority in the management of the patient with facial paralysis. The preoperative assessment of the facial paralysis patient is a critical component of their surgical management. Medical and surgical interventions should be used as appropriate to ensure ocular safety and health. Upper eyelid loading procedures are the gold standard for the surgical management of lagophthalmos in the setting of a paralyzed eye. Lower eyelid tightening can also be useful in restoring the aesthetics and function of the paralyzed eye. Irrespective of who manages the patient with facial paralysis, coordination of care between the ophthalmologist and the surgeon managing the patient with facial paralysis is critical.

REFERENCES

1. Sheehan JE. Progress in correction of facial palsy with tantalum wire and mesh. Surgery 1950;27:122.
2. Jobe R. A technique for lid loading in the management of the lagophthalmos of facial palsy. Plast Reconstr Surg 1974;53(1):29–32.
3. Anderson R, Gordy D. The tarsal strip procedure. Arch Ophthalmol 1979;97:2192–6.
4. Wobig J, Dailey R. Evaluation of the eyelids. In: Wobig J, Dailey R, editors. Oculofacial plastic surgery: face, lacrimal system and orbit. New York: Thieme; 2004. p. 30–3.
5. Wesley R. Management of facial palsy. In: Yen M, editor. Surgery of the eyelid, lacrimal system, and orbit. New York: Oxford University Press; 2012. p. 145–68.
6. Yu Y, Sun J, Chen L, et al. Lid loading for treatment of paralytic lagophthalmos [review]. Aesthetic Plast Surg 2011;35(6):1165–71.
7. Chung J, Yen M. Midface lifting as an adjunct procedure in ectropion repair. Ann Plast Surg 2007;59:635–40.

Static Facial Slings
Approaches to Rehabilitation of the Paralyzed Face

Morgan Langille, MD, FRCS(C)[a],*, Prabhjyot Singh, BSc, MD, MSc, FRCS(C)[b]

KEYWORDS

- Static facial slings • Facial paralysis • Allografts • Tensor fascia lata
- Percutaneous suture–based sling

KEY POINTS

- Facial paralysis is a physically and emotionally devastating condition for patients.
- Patients with facial paralysis benefit from cosmetic and functional improvement through the use of current facial rehabilitation techniques, including static facial rehabilitation.
- Static facial rehabilitation can be achieved through the use of autologous tissue grafts (tensor fascia lata), allografts (AlloDerm), synthetic grafts (Gore-Tex and expanded polytetrafluoroethylene), and permanent suspension sutures.
- A novel technique for midface suspension uses percutaneous suture–based slings.

INTRODUCTION: SURGICAL APPROACHES TO FACIAL PARALYSIS

Facial paralysis is a serious condition that can lead to significant cosmetic and functional impairment with a significant impact on the patient's quality of life. The causes for facial paralysis are widespread,[1] ranging from iatrogenic injury during surgical procedures to congenital conditions such as Moebius syndrome. Workup of patients with facial paralysis includes a detailed history, physical examination, and electrodiagnostic studies to evaluate any potential for return of facial nerve function. A longstanding facial nerve paralysis leads to significant facial asymmetry, leading to significant functional and social impairment. Complete facial nerve paralysis can affect various aspects of the forehead, eye, midface, mouth, and neck. Each of these anatomic locations can be treated either with procedures targeting the facial nerve or

with separate targeted surgical procedures to improve both cosmesis and function of a given area. There is a plethora of surgical procedures designed to address facial paralysis depending on the acuity of the paralysis and the anatomic structure being targeted.[2]

There are 2 types of surgical approaches to address facial paralysis. The first includes dynamic procedures that regain the ability of volitional movement of the face. Dynamic procedures involve restoring active movement and functionality to a paralyzed face, either through procedures to restore the function of an injured facial nerve or by restoring function with local or distant innervated muscle flaps.

Dynamic procedures involving free functional muscle transfer provide the opportunity for excellent functional rehabilitation outcomes of the paralyzed face. As an inherently more complex procedure, it has longer operative times and

Disclosure: The authors have nothing to disclose.
[a] Department of Surgery, Dalhousie University, Saint John Campus, Saint John, New Brunswick, Canada;
[b] Division of Otolaryngology - Head and Neck Surgery, Department of Surgery, The Scarborough Hospital, Toronto, Ontario, Canada
* Corresponding author. 1 Magazine Street, Unit 201, Saint John, New Brunswick E2K 5S9, Canada.
E-mail address: morgan.langille@gmail.com

Facial Plast Surg Clin N Am 24 (2016) 29–35
http://dx.doi.org/10.1016/j.fsc.2015.09.007
1064-7406/16/$ – see front matter © 2016 Elsevier Inc. All rights reserved.

higher intraoperative complication rates for high-risk patients compared with static rehabilitation techniques. Frail patients with extensive medical comorbidities may not be suitable candidates for free muscle transfer or other dynamic procedures. In some instances, dynamic procedures are not a viable option. Tumor ablation of the parotid or mastoid region may leave the patient with deficiencies in neurovascular structures or muscle that make dynamic procedures more difficult.[3]

The main goal of static rehabilitation of the paralyzed face is to improve facial symmetry and to improve static functions of the face, such as oral competence. Static facial procedures offer shorter surgical times and immediate results, but lack the ability to restore voluntary movement. Appropriately selected surgical procedures can improve facial symmetry and cosmesis either as an alternative to or in conjunction with dynamic procedures. Furthermore, dynamic rehabilitation does not address all aspects of facial symmetry, which are better addressed by static rehabilitation. For these reasons, static facial slings are an excellent surgical choice in a select subset of patients. Surgical procedures that allow for static rehabilitation of the midface are the focus of this article.

STATIC REHABILITATION OF THE PARALYZED MIDFACE

Patients with facial paralysis often have marked asymmetry of the midface, nasolabial fold, and mouth. This asymmetry creates cosmetic concerns that have been shown to adversely affect the patient's quality of life, and even cause psychological distress.[4] Patients who have facial paralysis are at a distinct disadvantage because they are unable to conceal their impairment, which often leads to social debilitation.[5] In addition, patients with marked asymmetry of the mouth may have poor oral competence, resulting in dysphagia and drooling with resultant poor functional outcomes. Correction of the midface offers patients improved cosmesis and functional outcomes. Preoperative examination, including facial asymmetry at full contraction and at rest, is vital for assessing the appropriate surgical technique and implant material. Surgical markings with the patient upright helps to reduce the effect of gravity intraoperatively for patients laying supine.

A static sling refers to a surgical technique that suspends the nasolabial fold and the oral commissure up to the region of the zygomatic arch and temporal fascia. There are 4 commonly described materials to provide the support: autologous tissue grafts, allografts, synthetic grafts, and permanent suspension sutures. The ideal implant is readily accessible, inexpensive, biocompatible, durable, predictable, easy to manipulate, and resistant to infection. However, none of the available grafts perform all of these functions perfectly, so the advantages and disadvantages of each choice must be weighed before selecting an implant for a particular patient. Besides the risk profile of a particular static sling, consideration of postoperative treatments such as radiation may influence the choice of static sling.[3] A brief description of different static sling options is given later.

Autologous Tissue Grafts

There are several options for autologous tissue grafts. The options range from the palmaris longus tendon[6] to the tensor fascia lata (TFL). TFL grafts have been successfully used to suspend the nostril, lips, lateral commissure, and lower eyelid.[7] The advantages of TFL and other autologous grafts include ease of harvest, predictable surgical outcomes, as well as abundant tissue to work with if harvested correctly. Autologous grafts have the benefit of transferring biological material from the same patient, therefore significantly decreasing the long-term risk of extrusion, infection, or rejection. The main disadvantages are increased surgical time and donor site morbidity. There is evidence that TFL grafts may undergo resorption postoperatively, but data are limited.[8] Several techniques have been described for the harvest of TFL. Minimally invasive techniques allow for harvest of the TFL through smaller incisions,[9] and newer techniques have described similar results without the use of specialized instruments.[10]

Synthetic Slings

Expanded polytetrafluoroethylene (ePTFE; more commonly known as Gore-Tex, Gore & Associates, Flagstaff, AZ), has been successfully used to address midface suspension in patients with facial paralysis. The main advantages of synthetic materials is that they are readily available, convenient, they shorten surgical time, and there is no donor site morbidity. The use of ePTFE as an implantable graft has been well documented, because it was initially used as a vascular graft.[11] It is microporous because of the structure of microfibrils, which allows greater biocompatibility and integration into host tissues. ePTFE is available in a variety of different sizes and thicknesses (1 mm and 2 mm), allowing reconstructive surgeons many choices when using different surgical approaches. Furthermore, ePTFE can easily be cut and trimmed intraoperatively to the exact size and shape required for a particular surgical result. ePTFE has been described as a reliable material to rehabilitate the midface.[12]

There are some disadvantages of using ePTFE for correction of midface asymmetry. ePTFE has been shown to stretch over time,[13] leading to relaxation of the desired surgical effect. An initial excellent correction may diminish with time, with worsening asymmetry as the stretching progresses. To counteract this relaxation, some investigators have suggested overcorrection. However, predicting the amount of relaxation has proved difficult and unreliable. Several studies have described prestretching at implantation, which can reduce this effect. However, even when prestretching is performed, it is still possible to have further stretching and failure of the surgical correction.[13]

Allografts

Allografts can overcome the disadvantages associated with autologous tissue grafts, such as prolonged operative time and donor site morbidity, but there is increased cost associated with the use of allografts. One of the most common allografts is acellular human dermis (AlloDerm, Lifecell Bridgewater, NJ). Acellular dermis is obtained by processing cadaveric dermis to remove all cellular elements. Its use has been described with excellent success rates for many applications in the head and neck,[14] from duraplasty[15] to repair of nasal septal perforations.[16] Acellular dermis is biocompatible because it has no remaining cellular material, minimizing the risk of reaction or inflammation. It has been used to suspend the midface and has a lower risk profile for infection and extrusion compared with synthetics, even in patients receiving radiation therapy.[17] AlloDerm has been shown to have no specific or minimal immune response, and it shows an affinity for ingrowth of host cells and possible revascularization.[3]

One of the disadvantages of acellular dermis is that it may stretch when put under tension,[8] which may necessitate revision surgical procedures. Its use also represents increased operative costs compared with autologous grafts. There has been some suggestion in the literature that acellular dermis may have a greater stiffness profile, and thus less relaxation over time, compared with ePTFE.[18]

SURGICAL TECHNIQUES

Various surgical techniques have been described to allow functional and cosmetic rehabilitation of the paralyzed face. These surgeries are designed for several areas of the face, including the forehead, periorbital area, midface, mouth, and nasolabial fold. Approaches to midface can include subcutaneous, sub–superficial musculoaponeurotic system (SMAS), and deep plane dissections, each of which offer surgeons different advantages in terms of operative time, complications, morbidity, as well as graft placement.[19] This article focuses specifically on the midface because the other techniques are described elsewhere.

Rhytidectomy

A standard rhytidectomy with plication or imbrication of the SMAS can provide an immediate improvement in facial symmetry of the midface. In the setting of long-standing facial paralysis, rhytidectomy alone leads to relapse of asymmetry in a short period of time. Rhytidectomy does not address the nasolabial folds to any great extent, and it does not improve oral competence in this patient population. For these reasons, rhytidectomy is typically used in conjunction with other surgical procedures for the management of patients with facial paralysis.

Autogenous fascia lata grafts are a popular therapeutic technique to improve facial symmetry either in conjunction with dynamic rehabilitation or as a stand-alone procedure. The fascia lata graft can be used to address different areas of the face, such as nostril suspension, bimalar suspension sling of the lower lip, lower eyelid suspension, lateral lip commissure, and platysmal transfer of the lower lip.[7]

Static Suspension Sling

A standard preauricular rhytidectomy incision may be extended inferiorly into the neck and can be used in combination with subciliary, nasolabial, and vermillion incisions to improve access to the midface for static procedures.[20] Access to the facial bony skeleton, specifically the zygomatic arch and zygomaticofacial suture line, is important to ensure adequate exposure for securing static slings.[3,21] The lower border placement of static slings often focuses on the upper and lower lip. Access to this area is achieved through vermillion border incisions that expose the orbicularis oris muscle.[3,21]

After selecting the desired graft material for a static sling, a tunnel is often created from the zygomatic region to the orbicularis oris muscle via several different approaches, most commonly the subcutaneous, sub-SMAS, or deep plane approaches mentioned earlier. The vector of pull is often considered to be in a posterior-superior direction from the vermillion/modiolus region to the zygomatic region. In addition to this, some investigators advocate a superior vector related to a subciliary incision or a nasolabial component.[21]

The selected graft can then be secured to the orbicular oris muscle or modiolus using either nonabsorbable sutures or long-dissolving sutures. These sutures are then attached to the selected graft material that has been tunneled to the zygomatic arch. The amount of correction is examined intraoperatively and a final length of the graft is selected, taking into consideration the relaxation profile of the graft selected.[3,21] The graft is then secured to the zygoma region using a variation of sutures, miniplates, and screws or Mitek anchors.[3,21,22]

Percutaneous Suture–Based Slings

A standard rhytidectomy alone allows for correction of facial asymmetry, but stretching of the SMAS causes effacement of the nasolabial fold, leaving a noticeable cosmetic difference compared with the nonparalyzed side. The nasolabial fold visually separates the cheek from the upper lip, creating an important static landmark. Surgical techniques designed to address only the position of the oral commissure and mouth often neglect to adequately recreate the nasolabial fold. A standard static sling surgical procedure requires a large incision at the oral commissure for placement and anchoring of the graft. Furthermore, a standard rhytidectomy and suspension sling can stretch, leading to a loss of the surgical correction. A novel procedure involving percutaneous suture–based slings has been described.[23] It is a hybrid procedure using a minimally invasive Gore-Tex strip along with percutaneously placed sutures to recreate a natural nasolabial fold.

With the patient awake and sitting upright, the desired nasolabial crease on the paralyzed side

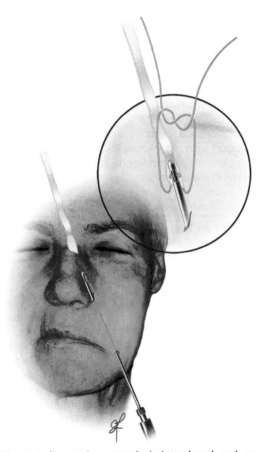

Fig. 1. A liposuction cannula is introduced and sutured to a Gore-Tex strip. (*From* Alam D. Rehabilitation of long-standing facial nerve paralysis with percutaneous suture-based slings. Arch Facial Plast Surg 2007;9(3):206; with permission; and *Courtesy of* CCF, 2006.)

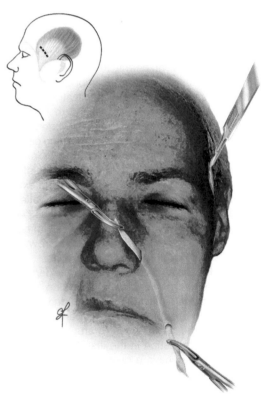

Fig. 2. The temporal incision is made and the Gore-Tex strip is clamped on each end. (*From* Alam D. Rehabilitation of long-standing facial nerve paralysis with percutaneous suture-based slings. Arch Facial Plast Surg 2007;9(3):206; with permission; and *Courtesy of* CCF, 2006.)

is marked out based on the measurements and location of the contralateral nonparalyzed side. The patient is then anesthetized and a laryngeal mask airway used. A small stab incision is made at each nasolabial crease and the oral commissure, 2 mm medial to the desired nasolabial crease. A liposuction cannula is used to create a tunnel in the subcutaneous plane between the 2 stab incisions (**Fig. 1**). This tunnel will form the new nasal labial crease. A thin (5 mm × 4 cm) Gore-Tex strip is then pulled through the subcutaneous tunnel. A hemostat is placed on each free end of the Gore-Tex strip to maintain the position of the implant during the percutaneous suturing.

The next step is to create a 2-cm to 3-cm incision in the temporal hair-bearing scalp on the ipsilateral side (**Fig. 2**). This incision will provide access for anchoring of the percutaneous sutures. Care is taken to dissect under the temporal parietal fascia, directly onto the deep temporal fascia, to preserve the integrity of the frontal branch of

the facial nerve if the patient regains facial nerve function.

A clear 4-0 Prolene suture (Ethicon Inc, Summerville, NJ) is then threaded on a 10-cm (4-inch) abdominal Keith needle to allow for passage from the temporal incision line down to the nasolabial fold. A micro–stab incision using a #11 blade is used in the new nasal labial fold, and the Prolene suture is passed from the temporal incision in the subcutaneous plane down to the micro–stab incision in the new nasolabial fold (**Fig. 3**). It is passed through the Gore-Tex implant twice to ensure proper anchoring of the suture. The suture is then passed back up to the temporal incision, and a retractor is used to protect the frontal branch of the facial nerve. This step is repeated until 4 or 5 suspension sutures are passed. Each individual suspension suture can be manipulated for appropriate tension to recreate the desired aesthetic appearance of the nasolabial fold. The sutures are then anchored to the deep temporal fascia using a Mayo needle (**Fig. 4**). The temporal

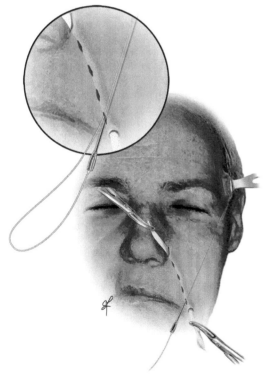

Fig. 3. The suture is passed through the implant, and out through the temporal incision. A retractor is used to protect the frontal branch of the facial nerve as the suture passes deep to it. (*From* Alam D. Rehabilitation of long-standing facial nerve paralysis with percutaneous suture-based slings. Arch Facial Plast Surg 2007;9(3):206; with permission; and *Courtesy of* CCF, 2006.)

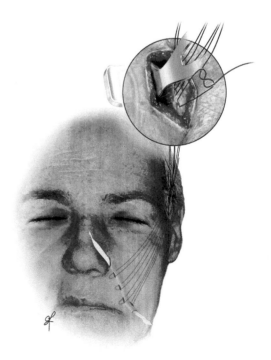

Fig. 4. The percutaneous sutures are anchored with a Mayo needle. (*From* Alam D. Rehabilitation of long-standing facial nerve paralysis with percutaneous suture-based slings. Arch Facial Plast Surg 2007;9(3):206; with permission; and *Courtesy of* CCF, 2006.)

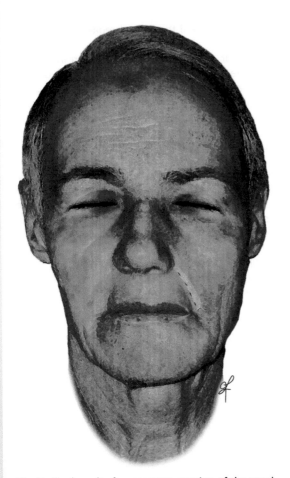

Fig. 5. Final result after recovery creation of the nasal labial fold using percutaneous sutures and Gore-Tex implant. (*From* Alam D. Rehabilitation of long-standing facial nerve paralysis with percutaneous suture-based slings. Arch Facial Plast Surg 2007;9(3):206; with permission; and *Courtesy of* CCF, 2006.)

incision is then closed, and the final result can be seen with an excellent recovery creation of the nasolabial fold (**Fig. 5**).

SUMMARY

Patients can expect an immediate result using static facial slings. Overcorrection may lead to a poor cosmetic appearance in the early stages; however, this is expected to improve once final stretching of the graft has been achieved. A new method using percutaneous suture–based slings is a short outpatient-based procedure that allows immediate and long-lasting correction of facial asymmetry in patients with facial paralysis.

REFERENCES

1. Melvin TA, Limb CJ. Overview of facial paralysis: current concepts. Facial Plast Surg 2008;24(2): 155–63.
2. Mehta RP. Surgical treatment of facial paralysis. Clin Exp Otorhinolaryngol 2009;2(1):1–5.
3. Winslow CP, Wang TD, Wax MK. Static reanimation of the paralyzed face with an acellular dermal allograft sling. Arch Facial Plast Surg 2001;3(1):55–7.
4. VanSwearingen JM, Cohn JF, Turnbull J, et al. Psychological distress: linking impairment with disability in facial neuromotor disorders. Otolaryngol Head Neck Surg 1998;118(6):790–6.
5. Macgregor FC. Facial disfigurement: problems and management of social interaction and implications for mental health. Aesthetic Plast Surg 1990;14(4): 249–57.
6. Toyserkani NM, Bakholdt V, Sørensen JA. Using a double-layered palmaris longus tendon for suspension of facial paralysis. Dan Med J 2015;61(3):1–5.
7. Rose EH. Autogenous fascia lata grafts: clinical applications in reanimation of the totally or partially paralyzed face. Plast Reconstr Surg 2005;116(1): 20–32 [discussion: 33–5].
8. Vural E, McLaughlin N, Hogue WR, et al. Comparison of biomechanical properties of Alloderm and Enduragen as static facial sling biomaterials. Laryngoscope 2006;116(3):394–6.
9. Bhatti AF, Soueid A, Baden JM, et al. Fascia lata harvesting: minimal access for maximum harvest. A new technique. Plast Reconstr Surg 2010;126(5): 277e–8e.
10. Tay VS, Tan KS, Loh IC. Minimally invasive fascia lata harvest: a new method. Plast Reconstr Surg Glob Open 2013;1(1):e6–7.
11. Soyer T, Lempinen M, Cooper P, et al. A new venous prosthesis. Surgery 1972;72(6):864–72.
12. Petroff MA, Goode RL, Levet Y. Gore-Tex implants: applications in facial paralysis rehabilitation and soft-tissue augmentation. Laryngoscope 1992; 102(10):1185–9.
13. Constantinides M, Galli SK, Miller PJ. Complications of static facial suspensions with expanded polytetrafluoroethylene (ePTFE). Laryngoscope 2001; 111(12):2114–21.
14. Shridharani SM, Tufaro AP. A systematic review of acelluar dermal matrices in head and neck reconstruction. Plast Reconstr Surg 2012;130(5 Suppl 2):35S–43S.
15. Bowers CA, Brimley C, Cole C, et al. AlloDerm for duraplasty in Chiari malformation: superior outcomes. Acta Neurochir (Wien) 2015;157(3):507–11.
16. Ayshford CA, Shykhon M, Uppal HS, et al. Endoscopic repair of nasal septal perforation with acellular human dermal allograft and an inferior

turbinate flap. Clin Otolaryngol Allied Sci 2003;28(1): 29–33.

17. Fisher E, Frodel JL. Facial suspension with acellular human dermal allograft. Arch Facial Plast Surg 1999;1(3):195–9.

18. Morgan AS, McIff T, Park DL, et al. Biomechanical properties of materials used in static facial suspension. Arch Facial Plast Surg 2004;6(5): 308–10.

19. del Campo AF. Update on minimally invasive face lift technique. Aesthet Surg J 2008;28(1):51–61 [discussion: 62].

20. Leckenby JI, Harrison DH, Grobbelaar AO, et al. Static support in the facial palsy patient: a case series

of 51 patients using tensor fascia lata slings as the sole treatment for correcting the position of the mouth. J Plast Reconstr Aesthet Surg 2014;67(3):350–7.

21. Konior RJ. Facial paralysis reconstruction with Gore-Tex soft-tissue patch. Arch Otolaryngol Head Neck Surg 1992;118(11):1188–94.

22. Biel MA. GORE-TEX graft midfacial suspension and upper eyelid gold-weight implantation in rehabilitation of the paralyzed face. Laryngoscope 1995; 105(8 Pt 1):876–9.

23. Alam D. Rehabilitation of long-standing facial nerve paralysis with percutaneous suture-based slings. Arch Facial Plast Surg 2007;9(3):205–9.

Temporalis Muscle Tendon Unit Transfer for Smile Restoration After Facial Paralysis

Kofi D. Owusu Boahene, MD

KEYWORDS

- Temporalis tendon transfer • Facial paralysis • Smile restoration • Facial reanimation

KEY POINTS

- The temporalis MTU procedure is an effective single-stage procedure for reanimating the paralyzed face and restoring smile.
- As with all functional muscle transfer procedures, surgeons performing the temporalis MTU procedure should be guided by the biomechanics of muscle function and the principles of tendon unit transfer muscle.
- Intraoperative electrical stimulation guides the establishment of the tension excursion relationship of the transposed tendon to guide optimal insertion to avoid overcorrection.

INTRODUCTION

Facial paralysis can be a devastating injury that results in functional impairment of the eyelids, nose, and lips. Impaired facial expression during communication and the associated blunted emotional exchange significantly affects the patient and their interactive circle and can lead to depression and strained relationships. Restoring facial tone, movement, and expression are primary goals of facial reanimation surgery and are achieved in almost all cases when the appropriate intervention is selected in a timely fashion. The functional end organ that produces dynamic movement consists of two discrete parts, the muscle belly and its tendinous attachment. An intact muscle tendon unit (MTU) with a given function may be repurposed to perform a new function by releasing and reattaching the tendon from its native insertion site to a new target. Functional MTU transfer is a common procedure performed in the upper extremity to restore hand function.

The temporalis tendon transfer procedure and digastric tendon transfer are examples of functional MTU transfer procedures used in the correction of facial paralysis. In 1952, McLaughlin[1] first introduced the concept and technique of mobilization and transposing the temporalis tendon for facial suspension. In the past two decades, the temporalis MTU transfer procedure has regained popularity as a single-stage option for reanimating the paralyzed face.[2,3] Although newer and refined techniques of free functional microvascular transfer of muscles, such as the gracilis, latissimus, pectoralis minor, and sternohyoid muscles flap, have added new dimensions to facial reanimation, tendon transfer remains a viable option in the management of facial paralysis.[4,5] The temporalis MTU originates from the temporal fossa as a broad fan-shaped muscle that converges into a tight tendon inserting on the coronoid process of the mandible. Detaching the temporalis muscle tendon from the coronoid process and inserting it into the upper lip can repurpose the temporalis muscle function for

Department of Otolaryngology Head and Neck Surgery, Johns Hopkins University School of Medicine, 601 North Caroline Street, Baltimore, MD 21878, USA
E-mail address: dboahen1@jhmi.edu

Facial Plast Surg Clin N Am 24 (2016) 37–45
http://dx.doi.org/10.1016/j.fsc.2015.09.004
1064-7406/16/$ – see front matter © 2016 Elsevier Inc. All rights reserved.

commissure contraction and smile restoration after facial paralysis. Understanding the functional anatomy of the temporalis muscle as an MTU and appropriately selecting patients for this procedure is a prerequisite for its successful application in facial reanimation. In addition, the principles and biomechanics of MTU function should guide the surgeon when applying the temporalis MTU for smile restoration.

INDICATIONS FOR TEMPORALIS TENDON TRANSFER

In 1974, Burkhalter[6] reported the indications for MTU in extremity injury, which are applicable to the temporalis tendon transfer: (1) the transfer can act as a substitute during regrowth of a nerve, which thereby reduces the time of function loss; (2) the transfer can act as a helper and add power to normal reinnervated muscle function; and (3) the transfer can act as a substitute when, statistically, the recovery after neurorrhaphy or nerve repair is poor. When presented with facial paralysis, the clinician should make the determination if the paralysis is reversible. Reversible paralysis is that which may recover spontaneously or after nerve repair or grafting. Timely nerve grafting or nerve substitution to reinnervate a reversibly paralyzed facial muscle yields superior results to muscle tendon procedures. Electromyogram studies in combination with clinical history can help establish the reversibility of the paralyzed facial muscle. In cases were the repaired nerve is expected to recover partially or slowly, the temporalis MTU procedure can be performed as an adjunct while waiting for regrowth of the nerve thereby reducing the time of facial dysfunction. A typical example is a patient who after a radical parotidectomy is scheduled to undergo postoperative radiotherapy. Although the facial nerve is grafted, a temporalis MTU can be performed at the same time to provide facial support. The temporalis MTU transfer procedure can also be considered as an option to upgrade partial recovery after facial paralysis. The indications for the temporalis MTU procedure overlap with those for free functional muscle transfer, such as the gracilis flap. Choosing between the temporalis MTU and the gracilis flap depends on individual patient features, patient desires, and the surgeon's expertise and success with either technique.

SURGICAL ANATOMY
Muscle Tendon Unit

The temporalis muscle is a fan-shaped muscle that originates from the temporal fossa, passes under the zygomatic arch, to insert on the coronoid process of the mandible. The muscle fibers are arranged more vertically anteriorly for elevation of the mandible and posterosuperiorly posteriorly for retraction of the mandible. Detailed examination of the muscle shows three clear parts: (1) the superficial part, (2) a zygomatic part, and (3) a deep part. The zygomatic part of the temporalis muscle originates from the zygomatic arch to insert into the superficial part of the temporalis as it inserts into the lateral surface of the coronoid process. The deep temporalis contains muscle bundles that originated from the temporal fossa along and inserts into the medial aspect of the coronoid process and retromolar triangle down to the buccinators line.[7]

Innervation

The muscle is innervated by the deep temporal nerves that arise from the mandibular division of trigeminal nerve and courses close to the mandibular condyle into the muscle. Typically, three deep temporal nerves corresponding to the anterior, middle, and posterior portions of the muscle are present. Intramuscularly, there is abundant intramuscular nerve fiber anastomosis from the anterior to posterior extent of the muscle.[8] Following the temporalis MTU procedure, voluntary movement for smile production requires that the patient clenches down on the affected side. Frequent practice with biofeedback and implementation of the acquired smile to social settings is necessary to improve the natural appearance of the temporalis smile.

Vascular Supply

The temporalis muscle is supplied by the anterior deep temporal artery, the posterior deep temporal artery, and the middle temporal artery. The arteries are situated on the medial (deep) aspect of the muscle and are medial to the coronoid process. Protecting the soft tissue surrounding the coronoid process during the coronoidectomy is important in preventing injury to these vessels.

PRINCIPLES AND BIOMECHANICS OF TEMPORALIS MUSCLE TENDON UNIT

The principles for MTU transfer have mostly resulted from experience in extremity surgery but are applicable in all situation of functional muscle transfer including the temporalis tendon transfer.[9] **Box 1** outlines the fundamental principles of MTU transfer procedures.

Box 1
The principles of tendon muscle unit transfer

The muscle selected as an MTU donor must be expendable and functioning

Adequate soft tissue bed for the transfer tendon

Full passive range of motion of the involved joints (no fixed deformity)

Adequate excursion and length of donor tendon

Direct line of pull

Suitable insertion technique and firm fixation

Synergy of transfer

Single function for each transferred tendon

The Selected Donor Muscle Must Be Expendable and Functioning

The success of muscle tendon transfer surgery depends on the proper selection of a donor muscle. First, the MTU selected as a potential donor must be expendable in that sacrificing its function should not cause significant morbidity. The temporalis muscle works in conjunction with the masseter muscle to raise the mandible during jaw closure. In the classic transfer of the temporalis muscle where a segment of the muscle is transposed over the zygomatic arch for facial suspension, residual temporalis muscle effect on the mandible is retained. In contrast, with orthodromic transfer of the temporalis MTU the effect of the temporalis muscle on the mandible is completely lost on the side of the transfer. Clinically, one or both temporalis tendons can be transferred without significant functional deficits as long as the medial pterygoids are intact.

The donor muscle selected for MTU transfer should also be functional. Muscles that have compromised function either from direct trauma, fibrosis, or partial denervation are not ideal donors for MTU transfer. The function of the temporalis muscle should be tested clinically by observing and palpating for contraction of the muscle in the temple area when the patient is asked to bite down. Intraoperatively, the temporalis muscle can also be stimulated with surface electrodes to detect contraction. Preoperative testing of the temporalis muscle function is particularly important in patients with multiple cranial nerve injuries, Möbius syndrome, or a history of previous cranial surgery where the temporalis muscle was divided. Patients who have previously undergone the traditional temporalis muscle transfer procedure may still be good candidates for the temporalis MTU procedure if strong contraction of the remnant muscle is elicited.

Muscles Selected for Transfer Should Have Adequate Strength and Excursion

The temporalis MTU is used to replace the function of upper lip elevators, mainly the zygomaticus major and minor muscle along a single vector of contraction. When replacing the function of a deficient muscle with that of a donor MTU, the donor muscle should have adequate strength and excursion that is comparable with that of the paralyzed muscle it is replacing. Choosing a donor MTU with contraction velocity similar to the muscle it is replacing is also desirable. The strength of a muscle depends on the maximal force it can generate. The maximal force of a muscle is proportional to its physiologic cross-sectional area and its excursion range to the length of the muscle fibers.[10] The length of the sarcomeres is a major determinant for force and excursion range. The speed of muscle fiber contraction is largely determined by the heavy chain of the myosin molecule that in turn determines the muscle type. Muscle fibers are traditionally classified into three groups depending on their physiologic behavior. Type I fibers are slow contracting, fatigue resistant, and generate small forces; type IIA fibers are fast contracting, fatigue resistant, and generate larger forces; and type IIB fibers are fast contracting, fatigue resistant, and generate the largest forces. Freilinger and colleagues[11] distinguished the function of the facial muscles based on the proportion of muscle fiber type. The muscles that attach to the oral commissure for lip elevation (zygomaticus major, levator labii superioris) are intermediate phasic muscles with a mixture of type I and type II fibers suited for sustained tone and fast phasic movement seen in facial expression. The temporalis muscle is made predominantly of type I fibers with about 13% of type II fibers.[12] This muscle fiber profile is adequate to maintain tone in the midface and generate the phasic contraction necessary from smile generation.

Suitable Soft Tissue Bed for Transfer

Muscles and their tendons are uniquely designed for smooth contraction and gliding by their myomysium, paratenon, and surrounding fat. For optimal contraction, MTUs should be transposed while maintaining these glide planes within a healthy soft tissue bed that is free from inflammation, edema, and scar. This is necessary to allow the tendon to glide freely untethered by adhesions and scar. The importance of an optimal soft tissue bed in MTU transfer has long been recognize as noted by Steindler[13] in 1919 who advocated for achieving soft tissue equilibrium, in which edema is resolved, joints are supple, and scars are soft, before proceeding with tendon transfer surgery. The temporalis tendon is commonly transposed through the buccal space to reach the oral commissure. Buccal fat pads should be preserved as soft tissue cushion that separated the transposed temporalis tendon from the surrounding muscles and bone. The buccal fat pad fills the masticator space and consists of a main body and four extensions: (1) buccal, (2) pterygoid, (3) superficial, and (4) deep temporal.[14] The deep temporal extension of the buccal fat pad lies directly over the temporalis muscle and its tendon separating it from the zygomatic arch. Disruption of the deep temporal fat pad risks scaring of the muscle fibers and tendon to zygomatic arch and disruption of its smooth contraction. The extension of the buccal fat pad into the buccal space passes anterior to the masseter and overlies the buccinator muscle as it courses to the lip musculature. The transposed temporalis tendon passes through the buccal extension to reach the melolabial crease and modiolus. To maintain a gliding path for optimal tendon movement, an adequate cushion of vascularized fat should be preserved on all sides of the tendon (**Fig. 1**).

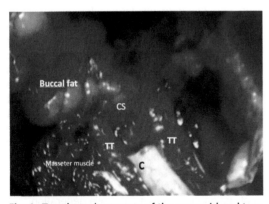

Fig. 1. Transbuccal exposure of the coronoid and temporalis tendon for coronoidectomy. The temporalis tendon (TT) is seen extending beyond the osteotomized coronoid segment (CS). Buccal fat is preserved to facilitate tendon gliding. The coronoid stump (C) may be reduced further to create space for tendon excursion and to minimize the chance of the osteotomized coronoid segments from restricting contraction or fusing back together structures including the zygomatic arch (*red*). At the ideal tension, the tendon is secured to the modiolus and lip margin.

There Should Be Full Passive Range of Motion of the Involved Lip

A temporalis tendon transfer procedure is less effective in restoring smile if the lip and oral commissure is stiff, scarred, and lacks passive movement. Scar and fibrosis around the lip, chin, and cheek that oppose the free excursion on the oral commissure can negatively affect the outcome of the temporalis tendon transfer. In burn patients, for example, stiff scarring around the lip renders restoration of dynamic excursion after MTU transfer less likely. The same may be true for postradiation cases when the fibrosis is extensive.[15] When present, these restrictive forces should be actively managed before the tendon transfer procedure.

Suitable Insertion Technique and Firm Fixation

A firm, stable, and gap-resistant fixation of the transposed temporalis tendon to orbicularis oris muscle and the modiolus is important. The importance of firm tendon fixation in MTU transfer is summarized by this statement by Strickland[16]: "It now seems irrefutable that the most effective method of returning strength and excursion to repaired tendons involves the use of strong, gap resistant suture techniques followed by the frequent application of controlled motion stress." Tendon dehiscence and fascia gaps are common reasons for failed temporalis tendon transfer procedures. In clinical practice, leaving a small piece of the coronoid attached to the temporalis tendon provides a stable platform for anchoring sutures. Holes may be drilled through the coronoid to allow firm suture placement. The orbicularis oris muscle around the modiolus is thin and atrophic in elderly patients and following prolonged paralysis. Fixating the temporalis tendon onto atrophic orbicularis oris muscles is prone to tendon disinsertion. In such cases, firm tendon fixation may be improved by first grafting fascia around the modiolus weeks to months before the temporalis MTU procedure.

Tension-Excursion Relationship of the Temporalis Muscle Tendon Unit

The biomechanical determinant of active muscle force after transfer is the classic Blix curve, which depicts the relationship between active force, passive force, and muscle length.[17] The sarcomere length–tension relationship shows that active muscle force increases as myofilament overlap increases. To achieve maximum force, the MTU must be set at the optimum sarcomere length–tension relationship for actin-myosin interaction. Freehafer and colleagues[18] suggested inserting the MTU as close as possible to its preoperative resting tension. Overstretching of the temporalis MTU results in low-active force generation. The routine practice of overcorrection to make up for anticipated slippage or stress relaxation may result in overstress and suboptimal excursion. Presently there are no widely available clinical tools for determining the ideal sarcomere length–excursion relationship to insert a transferred MTU. To determine an optimal length-tension of the transposed temporalis tendon, the muscle is stimulated intraoperatively once the tendon has been released to generate a tension excursion relationship. The average excursion of the temporalis tendon after its detachment from the mandible and stimulation at an optimized passive tension was 20.6 mm. Following tendon insertion, the mean oral commissure excursion was 15.5 mm.[19]

SURGICAL TECHNIQUE

The technical steps of the temporalis transfer procedure are straightforward once the concepts and pearls for optimizing dynamic excursion of the MTU are mastered. The main surgical steps include an approach to the coronoid process, tendon mobilization, and insertion. The procedure is commonly performed under general anesthesia. Neuromuscular blockade should be avoided to allow for muscle stimulation. Oral intubation with the tube sutured to the dentition avoids distortion of the lip. Transnasal intubation may also be used. The entire face should be prepared including the temporal scalp. Before bringing the patient to the operating room, the desired point of tendon insertion is determined based on the commissure contraction on the intact side in cases of unilateral paralysis.

Access Incision

Incision to access the buccal space and the coronoid may be external or transoral. In patients with deep melolabial folds, external melolabial incision may be used with the clear advantage of avoiding oral contamination. In younger patients and those with less defined melolabial creases, an intraoral incision placed under the lip provides wide exposure of the orbicularis muscle for tendon insertion and direct access to the buccal space and coronoid process. Intraoral incisions avoid facial scars but expose the surgical bed to oral contaminants, increasing the risk for infection. Placing a passive drain for a few days may be helpful.

Buccal Space Dissection

Dissection through the buccal space is mostly blunt and is facilitated by the use of malleable retractors. The parotid duct should be protected. Buccal fat should be preserved as a cushion against tendon scarring. As the malleable retractors are advanced deep the anterior edge of the mandibular ramus and the coronoid process are exposed.

Tendon Mobilization and Coronoidectomy

To protect the temporalis tendon from shredding, subperiosteal elevation of the fascia-periosteum tendon complex is performed on the medial aspect of the coronoid beginning from the retromolar area and extending superiorly to the level of the sigmoid notch. A Kocher is then placed on the coronoid and a right-angled hemostat passed between the coronoid bone and the elevated tendon into the sigmoid notch. The right angle hemostat acts as a retractor and as guide for coronoidectomy. It is important to keep a Kocher firmly secured on the coronoid before detaching the tendon to avoid retraction into the infratemporal fossa. A small reciprocating saw is used to osteotomize the coronoid. The tendon on the medial aspect of the coronoid is separated from any attachments to the medial pterygoid muscle and the lateral aspect from masseter muscle attachments (see **Fig. 1**). The remaining stump of coronoid process may be further shortened by removing additional bone to create space for tendon movement and to minimize the chance for fusion of the osteotomized segments. The tendon is then carefully freed laterally from the masseter muscle and medially from the medial pterygoid muscle. At this point the tendon is divided as low as possible for length and transposed through the buccal space toward the modiolus. If necessary, additional mobilization for length may be achieved by freeing the attachment of the temporalis muscle from the undersurface of the zygomatic arch. This is done carefully staying close to the undersurface of the zygomatic bone to preserve a fat layer between the arch and the muscle thereby preserving a fatty glide plane.

Generating a Tension-Excursion Relationship for the Temporalis Muscle Tendon Unit

After transposing the temporalis tendon through the buccal space toward the modiolus, a tension excursion relationship can be generated (**Fig. 2**). The temporalis muscle is electrically stimulated with transcutaneous or needle electrodes placed into the temporalis muscles. The DigiStim II plus stimulator (NeuroTechnology) commonly used by anesthesiologists may be used. With traction of the Kocher, the tension on the released tendon is manually varied while electrically stimulating the

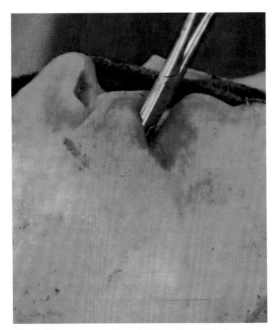

Fig. 2. Tension excursion relationship of the temporalis MTU determined in vivo with the aid of electrical stimulation. With a Kocher placed on the mobilized temporalis tendon, manual traction on the tendon is varied to alter the length of the temporalis MTU while stimulating the temporalis tendon. At the optimized length corresponding to the maximum force and excursion, a marker is placed on the Kocher to indicate the traction tension (length) at which to insert the temporalis MTU.

muscle. At the point of maximum force contraction a marker is placed on the Kocher clamp to represent the ideal traction tension and muscle length for maximal excursion. The marked Kocher is used to guide the degree of traction needed to ideally position the temporalis tendon for insertion. The tendon is then inserted at the determined optimal length (tension) based on the intraoperative excursion measurements.

Gaining Tendon Length

Fundamental to the temporalis MTU procedure is mobilization of the temporalis tendon from the mandible for reinsertion into the orbicularis oris muscle around the oral commissure. To gain tendon reach, Labbé described the temporalis tendon lengthening myoplasty procedure.[3] In his original description, the temporalis muscle is exposed through a scalp incision and the posterior third of the muscle released and elevated from its periosteal attachment. The zygomatic arch is osteotomized to gain access to the coronoid process for tendon release. By sliding the released muscle inferiorly, the muscle fibers are redistributed and

fixated inferiorly thereby allowing the released coronoid with the attached temporalis tendon to reach the lip. When releasing the temporalis muscle, care is taken to avoid injury to the neurovascular supply deep to the muscle. In addition, the released muscle should be refixated at the appropriate tension. Recent modifications by Labbé avoid osteotomy of the zygomatic arch and approach the coronoid through the buccal space similar to the minimally invasive temporalis tendon transfer procedure.[3] In a recent cadaveric analysis of the temporalis lengthening myoplasty procedure the authors catalogued seven steps in the procedure and quantified the potential length gained by each step. The median maximal total lengthening of all seven steps when performed together was 43.5 mm. The steps that contributed most to this lengthening were coronoidotomy and intraoral temporalis tendon dissection (median, 12.0 mm), incision of temporalis fascia insertion over the orbital rim (median, 6.5 mm), and zygomatic osteotomy with dissection of masseteric fibers (median, 11.5 mm).[20] The extent of incisions, dissection, and temporalis MTU mobilization described in the classic lengthening procedure disrupts the multiple glide planes at the level of the muscle belly and transition under the zygomatic arch, introduces external scars, but yields 4 cm or more of tendon transposition.

Tendon length may be gained by extension with fascia or donor tendon without mobilization of the muscle belly. The effect of tendon extension on muscle force was studied by Brunner.[21] The main disadvantage of tendon extension is the introduction of a passive noncontractile element (extra tendon/fascia) into a dynamic temporalis MTU system with the potential for reducing the effective contraction. The longer the tendon extension, the lesser is the contraction achievable. Therefore, the author does not recommend extensive (>2 cm) tendon extension.

Managing the Temporalis Tendon: to Lengthen or Not to Lengthen

Given the options available to gain tendon reach, it may be confusing when to select one method over another. First, the temporalis MTU should always be inserted close to its optimal passive length at which point there is maximal contraction. For optimal contraction overstretching should be avoided. Second, the temporalis MTU should be disturbed as little as possible to avoid scarring and disruptions of glide planes. Based on these principles, it is recommended to use intraoperative electrical stimulation and tension variation to help determine optimal length and tension at which to insert the mobilized tendon and the need for tendon lengthening. When the ideal tension is determined, if the tendon reaches the orbicularis oris muscle it is secured without extension. If the tendon at the optimal tension is within 1 to 2 cm of the orbicularis oris muscle, it is extended with fascia. When the tendon is more than 2 cm from the orbicularis oris muscle, the entire temporalis MTU should be released and advanced under the zygomatic arch toward the lip for insertion.

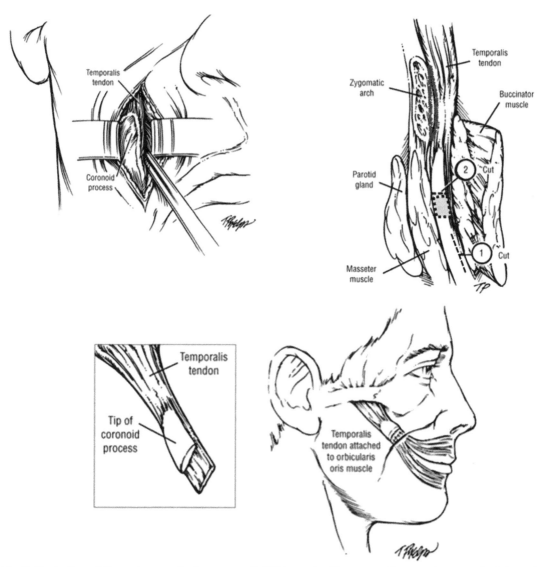

Fig. 3. Illustration of the major steps in the temporalis MTU transfer. The coronoid process is approached through the buccal space using either a melolabial crease incision or a sublabial incision. First a periosteal incision is made along the anterior edge of the mandibular ramus (*1*). The temporalis tendon wraps around the coronoid process but has an extension along the mandibular ramus down to the buccinator ridge. To gain adequate tendon length, subperiosteal tendon dissection should be performed toward the buccinator ridge. A coronoidectomy (*2*) is performed at the level of the sigmoid notch. Additional strip of bone (*yellow box*) may be removed to make room for the transposed MTU and to minimize interference and potential for fusion of the bone segment. Incremental tendon release and length is gained by freeing the MTU from surrounding tissue. (*Adapted from* Boahene KD, Farrag KD, Ishii L, et al. Minimally invasive temporalis tendon transposition. Arch Facial Plast Surg 2011;13(1):10; with permission.)

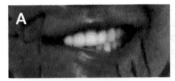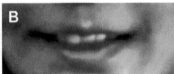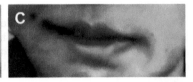

Fig. 4. Outcome after temporalis MTU transfer for right-sided congenital facial paralysis. The temporalis tendon was approached through an intraoral incision. Following coronoidectomy and tension excursion the relationship shows adequate length on the mobilized tendon for optimal insertion at the modiolus and orbicularis muscle. No tendon extension was necessary. (*A*) Asymmetric oral commissure excursion with asymmetric dental show. (*B*) Outcome with symmetric oral commissure excursion and dental show. (*C*) Isolated excursion of the right oral commissure with teeth clench.

Insertion Site

The upper lip elevators including the zygomaticus major insert and interdigitate with fibers of the orbicularis oris around the modiolus. The transposed temporalis tendon should be inserted as close to the lip margin as possible to mimic the insertion of the zygomaticus muscles. In this position, a natural melolabial fold develops and contraction of the temporalis muscle translates to movement of the mobile lip, dental show, and smile restoration. Insertion of the tendon in the melolabial fold results in a deep fold and muscle contractions that do not translate well into lip elevation.

Fig. 3 illustrates the major steps of the temporalis tendon transfer procedure.

Revision Temporalis Tendon Transfer

Common reasons to revise a failed temporalis tendon transfer procedure include lack of dynamic excursion and tendon disinsertion. Overcorrection and insertion of the tendon along the melolabial fold instead of the mobile lip are common reasons for inadequate excursion. When muscles have been inserted under excessive tension, structural and adaptive changes occur within the microstructure on the muscle fibers. These adaptive changes include rearrangement of sarcomere resulting in changes in contractile forces and the length-excursion relationship. In revision cases, the tendon should be exposed and isolated. Identifying the tendon within scar tissue may be challenging but is facilitated by electrical stimulation of the temporalis muscle. If the tendon was inserted along the melolabial fold, it should be mobilized, a tension excursion relationship should be determined, and the tendon reinserted along the lip margin with or without lengthening as described previously.

PHYSIOTHERAPY

Muscle is perhaps the most mutable of biologic tissues. After transfer of the temporalis tendon from the coronoid to the oral commissure, its mechanical properties change given the altered demands placed on muscle. Muscle-retraining exercises are therefore essential in optimizing the outcome of any muscle transfer procedure. In the preoperative period, patients visit a physical therapist who plans out specific exercises to strengthen the temporalis muscle and to identify isolated jaw movements that are essential in contracting the temporalis muscle. Patients should be motivated to direct their rehabilitation. After the first 2 postoperative weeks, active mobilization of the transposed temporalis MTU should be initiated. This should be followed by muscle-strengthening exercises. The main goal of the therapy is to systematically rehabilitate smile function by transferring labial functions to the transferred temporal muscle. Lambert-Prou[22] describes several phases of therapy to acquire a temporal smile. The first phase, termed the mandibular smile, involves mobilization of the mandible by contraction of the transferred temporalis muscle and inducing an elevation of the oral commissure. The second phase, the voluntary temporal smile, is attained by contracting of the temporalis muscle without mandibular movement, which remains under voluntary control. The smile produced should become as symmetric as possible (**Fig. 4**). Finally, the last phase focuses on achieving a spontaneous smile independent of mandibular movement, called spontaneous temporal smile. Biofeedback methods are helpful in this process. The role of electrical stimulation is unclear. As demonstrated by Coulson and colleagues,[23] repeated exercises and practice with the aid of video feedback loops of the best symmetric smile are powerful tools to achieve a spontaneous smile adapted for social settings.

SUMMARY

The temporalis MTU is a power technique for restoring facial tone, symmetry, and smile after facial paralysis. Guided by the principles and biomechanics of muscle contraction surgeons can reliably reanimate the paralyzed face using the temporalis tendon transfer procedure. Intraoperative assessment with electrical stimulation to determine the tension-excursion relationship of the MTU is necessary to improve the outcome. Overcorrection should be avoided by lengthening the tendon when the tendon deficiency is less than 2 cm or by advancement of the entire temporalis MTU when the tendon deficiency is larger.

REFERENCES

1. McLaughlin CR. Surgical support in permanent facial paralysis. Plast Reconstr Surg 1953;11:302–14.

2. Labbé D, Huault M. Lengthening temporalis myoplasty and lip reanimation. Plast Reconstr Surg 2000;105(4):1289–97.

3. Boahene KD, Farrag TY, Ishii L, et al. Minimally invasive temporalis tendon transposition. Arch Facial Plast Surg 2011;13(1):8–13.

4. Manketlow R. Free muscle transplantation for facial paralysis. Clin Plast Surg 1984;11:2–5.

5. Alam DS, Haffey T, Vakharia K, et al. Sternohyoid flap for facial reanimation: a comprehensive preclinical evaluation of a novel technique. JAMA Facial Plast Surg 2013;15(4):305–13.

6. Burkhalter WE. Early tendon transfer in upper extremity peripheral nerve injury. Clin Orthop Relat Res 1974;(104):68–79.

7. Sedlmayr JC, Kirsch CF, Wisco JJ. The human temporalis muscle: superficial, deep, and zygomatic parts comprise one structural unit. Clin Anat 2009; 22(6):655–64.

8. Wisco J, Cantelmi D, Davies J, et al. Temporalis muscle innervation patterns are generally conserved across subjects. FASEB J 2011;25:872.4.

9. Boahene KD. Principles and biomechanics of muscle tendon unit transfer: application in temporalis muscle tendon transposition for smile improvement in facial paralysis. Laryngoscope 2013;123(2):350–5.

10. Lieber RL. Skeletal muscle architecture implications for muscle function and surgical tendon transfer. J Hand Ther 1993;6:105–13.

11. Freilinger G, Happak W, Burggasser G, et al. Histochemical mapping and fiber size analysis of mimic muscles. Plast Reconstr Surg 1990;86(3):422–8.

12. Korfage JAM, Van Eijden TMGJ. Regional differences in fibre type composition in the human temporalis muscle. J Anat 1999;194(Pt 3):355–62.

13. Steindler A. Operative treatment of paralytic conditions of the upper extremities. J Orthop Surg 1919; 1:608–24.

14. Stuzin JM, Wagstrom L, Kawamoto HK, et al. The anatomy and clinical applications of the buccal fat pad. Plast Reconstr Surg 1990;85(1):29–37.

15. Griffin GR, Abuzeid W, Vainshtein J, et al. Outcomes following temporalis tendon transfer in irradiated patients. Arch Facial Plast Surg 2012;14(6):395–402.

16. Strickland JW, editor. The hand: master techniques in orthopaedic surgery. Philadelphia: Lippincott-Raven; 1998.

17. Gordon AM, Huxley AF, Julian FJ. The variation in isometric tension with sarcomere length in vertebrate muscle fibers. J Physiol 1966;184:170–92.

18. Freehafer AA, Peckham HP, Keith MW. Determination of muscle tendon unit properties during tendon transfer. J Hand Surg Am 1979;4:331–9.

19. Boahene KD, Ishii LE, Byrne PJ. In vivo excursion of the temporalis muscle-tendon unit using electrical stimulation: application in the design of smile restoration surgery following facial paralysis. JAMA Facial Plast Surg 2014;16(1):15–9.

20. Moubayed SP, Labbé D, Rahal A. Lengthening temporalis myoplasty for facial paralysis reanimation. An objective analysis of each surgical step. JAMA Facial Plast Surg 2015;17(3):179–82.

21. Brunner R. Changes in muscle power following tendon lengthening and tendon transfer. Orthopade 1995;24(3):246–51.

22. Lambert-Prou MP. The temporal smile. Speech therapy for facial palsy patients after temporal lengthening myoplasty. Rev Stomatol Chir Maxillofac 2003;104(5):274–80 [in French].

23. Coulson SE, Adams RD, O'Dwyer NJ, et al. Physiotherapy rehabilitation of the smile after long-term facial nerve palsy using video self-modeling and implementation intentions. Otolaryngol Head Neck Surg 2006;134(1):48–55.

The Gracilis Free Flap

Babak Azizzadeh, MD[a],*, Kelly J. Pettijohn, MD[b]

KEYWORDS

- Facial reanimation • Gracilis muscle free flap • Technique • Anatomy • Outcomes

KEY POINTS

- The neurovascular pedicle of the gracilis free flap is composed of a single arterial branch arising most commonly from the adductor branch of the profunda femoris, two vena comitantes, and the obturator nerve.
- Numerous neural sources have been used in combination with the gracilis flap, including the masseteric, hypoglossal, spinal accessory, and phrenic nerves. A cross-face nerve graft that uses a functioning contralateral facial nerve branch allows for the greatest degree of emotive and spontaneous reanimation.
- A 2-stage procedure involving a cross-face nerve graft in stage 1 and, after axonal regeneration has occurred, a gracilis free flap in stage 2, has been found to be highly successful in dynamic reanimation.
- In patients with paralysis of less than 2 years duration, cranial nerve substitution should be considered in stage 1 to decrease atrophy of the facial musculature.
- Outcomes using the described 2-stage procedure are excellent, with a low flap failure rate and significant improvement in facial symmetry/smile excursion; however, it is not uncommon for patients to require a third stage to refine the flap.

INTRODUCTION

Facial paralysis is a devastating condition that often results in significant negative social and psychological outcomes.[1] Demonstrating the social value on facial expression, Sinno and colleagues[2] found that healthy individuals would be willing to sacrifice 8 years of life and undergo a surgery associated with 21% mortality to correct a facial paralysis. Certainly, optimal recovery of facial function can be achieved when immediate neurorrhaphy of a freshly transected nerve is performed; however, this is often not feasible due to the etiology of paralysis. Ideal treatment of a unilateral facial paralysis not amenable to direct repair would restore resting tone/bulk and would allow for symmetric, spontaneous, and dynamic function.

Smile, although a very important aspect of facial expression, is not the only endpoint in rehabilitation. Normal social interaction relies on our ability to react to conversation with subtle facial expression changes. In addition to smile, re-creation of such subtle facial movements is the ultimate goal in facial reanimation.

Free-tissue transfer has afforded a modality of restoring bulk, dynamic function, and spontaneity, with the gracilis free flap presently leading as the gold-standard donor muscle. In this article, we focus on the gracilis free flap as it is used in dynamic facial reanimation. We discuss a 2-staged treatment used by the senior author (BA) that achieves optimal restoration of resting tone and spontaneous movement.

Disclosure Statement: The authors have no relevant disclosure to this topic.
[a] Department of Head and Neck Surgery, University of California, Los Angeles, 9401 Wilshire Boulevard #650, Westwood, Beverly Hills, CA 90212, USA; [b] Department of Head and Neck Surgery, David Geffen School of Medicine at UCLA, 10833 Le Conte Avenue, CHS 62-237, Westwood, Los Angeles, CA 90095-1624, USA
* Corresponding author.
E-mail address: drazizzadeh@gmail.com

facialplastic.theclinics.com

HISTORY

Following the advent of free-tissue transfer, the gracilis muscle was identified as a useful source of tissue for reconstruction of small traumatic or iatrogenic defects. Its utility was based on its relative accessory function in leg adduction, consistent anatomy, and comparative ease of harvest. Transplantation of the gracilis muscle was first described in 1952 by Pickrell and colleagues,[3] who used the muscle for rectal sphincter reconstruction. In the 1970s, Harii and colleagues[4] were the first to use the gracilis free flap in the head and neck, using it to reconstruct traumatic and iatrogenic temporal defects with successful outcomes. Harii and colleagues[5] subsequently went on to use the flap for dynamic reanimation of facial paralysis, using the deep temporal nerve for neurotization. This method of reinnervation allowed for smile via a voluntary bite action; however, the results appeared overexaggerated and the smile was not, by design, spontaneous (**Fig. 1**).[5]

O'Brien later used a 2-stage, cross-facial nerve graft (CFNG) technique with a gracilis free flap. The cross-facial approach was based on the method pioneered by Thompson and Gustavoson, in which a CFNG was sutured to the distal buccal branches of the unaffected facial nerve and anastomosed with the motor nerve of an extensor digitorum brevis free flap on the paralyzed side.[6] Using the gracilis flap and a CFNG, O'Brien and colleagues[7] found a 51% success rate in a cohort of 62 patients. Although their early work demonstrated mixed results, their technique established a starting point in dynamic reanimation using the gracilis flap.

ALTERNATE DONOR SITES

In the late 1980s, interest in dynamic facial reanimation grew, and a number of other donor sites for free-muscle transfer were explored. The pectoralis minor, serratus anterior, latissimus dorsi, extensor digitorum longus, rectus femoris, and rectus abdominis were all studied as potential donor muscles in dynamic facial reanimation.[8–13] Of these, the gracilis, pectoralis minor, and latissimus dorsi have demonstrated the greatest success.

Harrison and Grobbelaar[14] published the results of 637 patients treated for unilateral facial paralysis with pectoralis minor free-muscle transfers between 1981 and 2008. Their experience found that 354 had an excellent outcome, as assessed by the operating surgeon; 27.2% required revision

procedures, and 13.3% had delayed tightening of the muscle.

The latissimus dorsi has also been demonstrated as a fair candidate for dynamic facial reanimation. Takushima and colleagues[15,16] published results of their 1-stage latissimus dorsi muscle transfer, whose success may approach that of the gracilis flap. In this report, 87% of cases demonstrated muscle contraction in analysis of 351 transfers. Their group also noted that the latissimus dorsi provides the optional use of an overlying skin paddle, which can be beneficial in reanimation after ablative procedures. The bulk of this flap, however, does limit its utility in nonablative reanimation.

Despite the plethora of described donor sites, new candidates for free-muscle transfer are still under investigation. Alam and colleagues[17] recently published preclinical results of cadaveric evaluation of the sternohyoid muscle. Their findings demonstrated that the superior thyroid artery is reliable as the vascular pedicle for this novel flap. Given the length of the motor nerve (the ansa cervicalis), which could allow for a single-stage procedure, the thin muscle caliber, and nonessential endogenous function, this muscle could represent an excellent candidate for reanimation in the future, pending further clinical evaluation.

At the present time, the gracilis free flap is the gold standard for free-tissue facial reanimation. Its thin bulk, contractile strength, reliable pedicle anatomy, and low donor-site morbidity make it an ideal donor site in dynamic reanimation.

ANATOMY

The gracilis muscle is one of the adductors of the leg, located in the medial thigh. It is the most superficial of all of the medial thigh muscles. It originates from the ischiopubic ramus and inserts onto the medial tibia below the condyle via the pes anserinus. On average, the muscle measures approximately 25 cm in length. Owing to its name, based on the Latin word *gracile,* meaning slender, it is straplike and thin, tapering from superior to inferior from approximately 6 cm to 4 cm. At its insertion, it is located posteromedial to the adductor longus (**Fig. 2**). This muscle and its tendinous insertion are readily palpable, thereby facilitating identification of the gracilis muscle.

A single arterial branch arising most commonly from the adductor branch of the profunda femoris comprises the arterial supply to the proximal muscle in 73% to 87% of patients.[18,19] The vessel is on average 1.6 mm in diameter.[19] Infrequently, the arterial supply can alternatively be found to arise

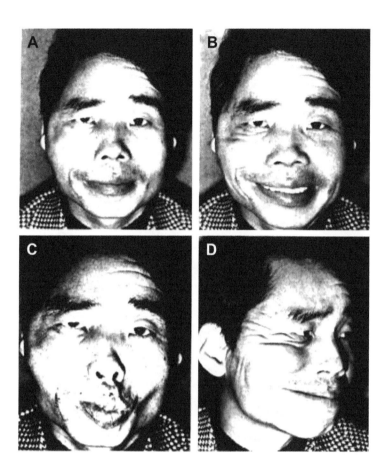

Fig. 1. Results from early dynamic reanimation using the gracilis free flap by Harii and colleagues in 1976. The motor nerve of the gracilis muscle was anastomosed to the deep temporal branch of the mandibular nerve (V3). In this configuration, smile is generated with voluntary bite action. (*A*) Results 8 months postoperatively at rest and (*B*) with smile. (*C*) Pucker motion and (*D*) full smile generated with bite action. Results were exaggerated with smile and somewhat weak at rest. (*From* Harii K, Ohmori K, Torii S. Free gracilis muscle transplantation, with microneurovascular anastomoses for the treatment of facial paralysis: a preliminary report. Plast Reconstr Surg 1976;57(2):141; with permission.)

from the medial circumflex artery or combination of both of these arteries. The vascular pedicle is found entering the undersurface of the proximal third of the muscle after passing between the adductor longus and brevis. Its entry point is typically 8 to 10 cm below the pubic tubercle. Two vena comitantes draining into the deep leg venous system can be found running with the artery.[20]

The muscle is innervated by the anterior branch of the obturator nerve, which can measure up to 12 cm in length. It is typically found approximately 6 cm from the pubic tubercle.[19] The motor nerve often divides into branches innervating the superior and inferior muscle separately. This division can be used for division of 2 functioning units.[21]

NERVE SELECTION FOR NEUROTIZATION

Beginning with Harii and his use of the deep temporal branch of the mandibular division of the trigeminal nerve, a number of modalities for neural power in free-tissue transfer have been described. Selection of the appropriate nerve for innervation

of the gracilis free-tissue transfer hinges on patient goals and the etiology of paralysis.

In the 1970s, the CFNG was developed by Smith[22] and Scaramella,[23] using an intact contralateral facial nerve for innervation of the paralyzed side. The goal of such a technique was to attain synchronized and spontaneous movement in the case of unilateral paralysis. Initially, this methodology was used in an effort to neurotize the endogenous paretic muscles, but was found to be limited in its success should more than a few months elapse between onset of paralysis and neurotization.[24] Although its use in this regard may have been limited, it was later applied to free-tissue transfer, initially in a 1-stage procedure in which the CFNG was placed in the same procedure as the free-tissue transfer. The process was later modified to a 2-stage procedure, which is most commonly used today.[7]

Compared with other neural sources, the use of the CFNG in combination with a gracilis free flap allows for the greatest degree of spontaneity in facial expression, and is the preferred methodology for neurotization by the senior author (BA). The senior

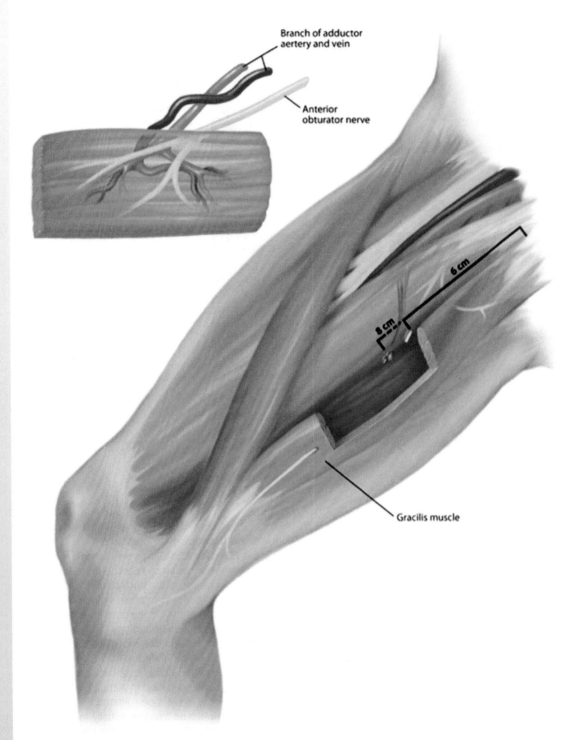

Fig. 2. The vascular pedicle to the gracilis muscle most commonly arises from branches of the adductor artery and vein. This is typically located 8 to 10 cm below the pubic tubercle. The anterior branch of the obturator nerve, which can be up to 12 cm in length, is typically found near the vascular pedicle, but can be as low as 15 cm below the pubic tubercle. (*Courtesy of* B. Azizzadeh MD, Beverly Hills, CA.).

author (BA) uses a 2-stage procedure. In the first stage, a sural nerve graft is tunneled from the zygomatic branch of the intact facial nerve to the contralateral gingivobuccal sulcus. Six to 9 months is allowed for axonal regrowth, and thereafter, the nerve graft is anastomosed to the obturator nerve of the gracilis in the second stage. Technical aspects of the procedure are described in more detail later in this article.

In recent years, a single-stage procedure wherein the obturator nerve is directly tunneled across the upper lip and connected to the contralateral facial nerve has been studied. Although it does have the benefit of the decreased morbidity of a second procedure, and similar to the 2-stage procedure, allows for spontaneous facial expression, it was found to have a decreased degree of symmetry at rest, and thus, is thought to have a less favorable result.[25]

Of course, not all patients have an available contralateral facial nerve, as is the case in Mobius syndrome (congenital absence of bilateral facial nerves). In such patients, a CFNG is not a viable option. The nerve to the masseter is the most commonly used source of reinnervation in such patients. As compared with the CFNG, this neural source does not allow for the same degree of spontaneity, given that generation of smile depends on a conscious bite action; however, it has been found to allow for a greater degree of excursion of the oral commissure compared with the CFNG.[26,27] Additionally, there are studies that report that most patients are able to develop some degree of spontaneous smile over time due to cortical plasticity.[28] Dual innervation with CFNG and masseteric nerve is being currently studied at several centers.

Other neural sources, such as the phrenic, spinal accessory, and hypoglossal nerve, have also been attempted. These nerves are not commonly used given the high donor site morbidity (hemitongue atrophy/deviation in the case of the hypoglossal and trapezius atrophy in the case of the spinal accessory nerve). Moreover, significant voluntary movement is required to generate facial expression with the use of these neural sources.[29]

PATIENT SELECTION

Numerous traumatic, malignant, congenital, iatrogenic, and infectious etiologies can result in facial paralysis. A clear delineation of mechanism of paralysis is critical in development of a treatment plan. Traumatic or iatrogenic facial nerve injury to the distal branches of the facial nerve may be amenable to a direct end-to-end anastomosis if identified quickly, and this approach affords the best outcome. Ideally, direct repair would take place within 3 days, before axon degeneration, which allows for the use of a nerve stimulator for identification of the distal branches, but in general, the longer the delay in repair, the worse the outcome on facial function.[30,31]

Duration of symptoms is also critical, as patients with paralysis from Bell Palsy may continue to improve as much as a year or more from onset. Before this time, such patients should not be offered reanimation. Patients with paralysis related to a parotid or temporal bone malignancy with large surgical defects and/or a history of radiation therapy to the area are not typically offered CFNG/free muscle transfer due to limited outcomes in the setting of a previously operated/irradiated surgical field. These patients are advised to undergo orthodromic temporalis tendon transfer by the senior author (BA).[32]

In cases of complete paralysis not amenable to direct repair or otherwise thought to be unlikely to recover, the patient should be considered a candidate for reanimation. The senior author proposes a treatment plan based on classification of patients into 1 of 4 groups according to etiology and duration of paralysis (summarized in **Table 1**).

Severe/Complete Paralysis Less Than 2 Years

Individuals who develop acute paralysis secondary to intracranial tumors or temporal bone fracture, in which the proximal branch of the facial nerve is not accessible, are amenable to cranial

---

Table 1
Treatment strategy by patient group

Severe/Complete paralysis <2 y	Two-stage cross-facial nerve graft (CFNG)/gracilis free muscle transfer Nerve substitution procedure at first stage
Severe/Complete paralysis >2 y	Two-stage CFNG/gracilis free muscle transfer
Partial paralysis with Synkinesis	Selective neurectomy of the lower division facial nerve; possible 2-stage CFNG/gracilis free muscle transfer
Bilateral paralysis	One-stage masseteric nerve to gracilis free muscle transfer or Bilateral orthodromic temporalis tendon transfer

nerve substitution techniques with the coaptation of the distal trunk of the facial nerve to the hypoglossal or masseteric nerves.[33–35] It is critical that the facial nerve injury is deemed permanent and complete before embarking on these procedures, as they require transection of the facial nerve distal to the stylomastoid foramen. Furthermore, it is crucial that the procedure is undertaken less than 2 years after the facial nerve paralysis to ensure that the facial musculatures have not developed permanent atrophy.[36] Cranial nerve substitution techniques do an excellent job of restoring tone and providing dynamic reanimation. The smile mechanism, however, is not spontaneous, requiring extensive retraining and can also result in significant synkinesis. The senior author often combines cranial nerve substitution techniques with CFNG and secondary gracilis flap to improve resting tone and restore spontaneous smile mechanism.[36–38]

Severe/Complete Paralysis Greater Than 2 Years

Long-standing unilateral paralysis has also been observed to have success with CFNG and second-stage gracilis flap; however, due to the duration of paralysis and long-term atrophy, these patients are unlikely to improve bulk/tone with an additional cranial nerve substitution procedure.

Partial Paralysis with Synkinesis

Patients with partial paralysis often suffer from synkinesis, in which the simultaneous contraction of the facial muscles can result in activation of contradictory muscles, thereby causing an "auto-paralysis," in which patients may be unable to generate a meaningful smile. These patients are unlikely to benefit from an additional nerve substitution (ie, XII-VII procedure), as they have not experienced denervation and atrophy of the facial muscles. In the senior author's practice, such patients are treated with botulinum toxin, neuromuscular retraining, and selective neurectomy of the lower division of the facial nerve. Some severely affected individuals may also benefit from a 2-stage CFNG with gracilis free tissue transfer.

Bilateral Paralysis

Bilateral facial nerve paralysis is rare, seen in only 1.5% of affected patients. Etiology is most commonly congenital, autoimmune, or infectious.[39] In patients who do not have a functional contralateral facial nerve, as is the case in infectious bilateral paralysis or Mobius syndrome, among others, there are no functional branches of the facial nerve to use for CFNG. Therefore,

reanimation in these patients is carried out in a single-single stage procedure using the masseteric branch of mandibular nerve. The result is less natural, requiring the patient to bite down to generate a smile. There is no spontaneity to facial expression, as all movement must be voluntarily generated. This article focuses on CFNG using the zygomatic branch of the facial nerve in cases of unilateral paralysis. For further details regarding masseteric nerve innervation in free tissue transfer, refer to publications by Manktelow and colleagues.[28]

TECHNICAL CONSIDERATIONS

Appropriate patient selection is the critical first step in a successful outcome of a 2-stage free tissue transfer, including consideration of a cranial nerve substitution procedure in patients with a complete facial paralysis for less than 2 years (see section "Patient selection"). The various donor muscles and neurotization options were discussed previously, and the subsequent sections will describe the technical aspects of a 2-stage gracilis muscle flap innervated by a CFNG, which is the preferred technique of the senior author (BA) due to its optimal restoration of spontaneous facial expression, resting facial tone, and capacity for emotive facial expression.

Stage I: Cross-Face Nerve Grafting

General endotracheal anesthesia is induced and the patient is prepped and draped in the standard fashion, exposing the lower leg from knee to ankle with the lateral malleolus oriented upward and the entire face from the postauricular hairline of the unaffected side to the contralateral postauricular hairline. Anesthesia should be informed that nerve monitoring will be used and, thus, paralysis should be avoided. The procedure begins with harvest of the sural nerve graft by making a 2-cm incision approximately 1.5 cm posterior and 2.0 cm superior to the lateral malleolus. The nerve is then identified after minimal dissection through the subcutaneous tissues. Dissection of the nerve is carried distally 2 to 3 cm. At this point, the nerve is transected and a retracting 2 to 0 silk suture is placed. The nerve is placed into a tendon stripper, which is then used to dissect the nerve 10 to 20 cm superiorly in the direction of the popliteal fossa through the single incision. Transverse stair-step incisions could be utilized until the surgeon is comfortable with the single-incision technique. Endoscopic approaches have also been described using a single incision but are not utilized due to prohibitive costs of equipment.[40] The sural nerve graft is then harvested and the leg incision is closed in the usual fashion.

Attention is then turned to the inset of the nerve graft. Facial nerve monitors are placed in the orbicularis oris and at the oral commissure; 1:100,000 epinephrine can be used for vasoconstriction, but lidocaine should be avoided given its inhibitory effect on nerve stimulation. A pre-auricular incision is made from the temporal tuft to the inferior aspect of the lobule. A 5-cm skin flap is raised and the superficial musculoaponeurotic system (SMAS) is incised from the angle of the mandible to the medial aspect of the zygomatic arch, taking care to avoid the frontal branch of the facial nerve, and dissection is continued deep to the SMAS. In this plane, the zygomatic branch of the facial nerve is identified beneath the masseteric fascia using nerve stimulation. It is important that the selected branch does not also cause eye closure, as this can result in synkinesis of the gracilis muscle.

While keeping the orientation of the sural nerve intact, the proximal (nontagged) end of the nerve is loaded into the plastic end of a drain with a trochar using a 4 to 0 Prolene suture. The nerve graft will ultimately be placed in its reverse direction, as it is a sensory nerve, and this direction will allow for axon regeneration. The trochar is then pushed through the surgical field to the midline gingivobuccal sulcus, leaving the distal (tagged) end of the nerve near the selected zygomatic branch and the trochar is removed. The nerve is then tagged with a Prolene and hemoclip within the submucosal pocket. The previously identified zygomatic branch is anastomosed to the sural nerve with 9 - 0 nylon suture. The gingivobuccal incision is closed. In a layered fashion with minimal tension, the SMAS, deep dermal, and dermal layers are closed. Please see the article by Kelly and colleagues elsewhere in this issue for more detailed and alternative description of the CFNG procedure. For further details, please reference a recent publication on the CFNG.[41]

Stage II: Gracilis Free Muscle Transfer

Nerve regeneration from the CFNG is expected at a rate of 1 to 2 mm per day.[42] Following a 4-month to 6-month delay, the nerve is examined for a positive Tinel sign, which signifies that axonal regrowth has occurred. At this point, the patient is ready for transfer of the gracilis flap. The patient is prepped and draped in the usual sterile fashion, exposing the pubic symphysis and the medial condyle of the femur. Under general anesthesia, the procedure begins with biopsy of the sural nerve graft to confirm nerve regrowth.

Attention is then turned to harvest of the flap. The contralateral gracilis muscle (with respect to the facial paralysis) is ideally harvested, as it allows for greater ease of inset due to the location of the recipient/donor vessels. At a point 3 to 4 cm below the pubic symphysis, a longitudinal incision is made between the adductor tubercle and the medial condyle of the femur, 10 to 15 cm in length. The incision is carried down to the muscular fascia, and the gracilis muscle is identified. The adductor longus is identified and retracted superiorly (**Fig. 3**). With a slight posterior retraction of the gracilis muscle, the neurovascular anatomy can be identified arising from the underbelly of the proximal portion of the adductor longus muscle. The obturator nerve is typically 1 to 2 cm superior to the vascular pedicle. The dissection along the neurovascular pedicle is extended to the desired length.

Measurements of the desired flap dimensions are taken. The distance between the oral commissure and temple is typically used as an approximate length of muscle. The width is dependent on the age of the patient and body habitus. Approximately one-third to one-half of the medial aspect of the gracilis muscle is harvested after the resting position of the muscle is marked, such that the native length of the muscle can be re-established at inset. The resultant muscle may need to be further debulked to achieve a weight of 10 to 30 g, depending on the size of the patient (**Fig. 4**). The debulked muscle edges are lightly cauterized to reduce hematoma risk. The superior and inferior edges of the muscle are transected using a GIA stapler (Covidien, Irvine, CA, USA) creating a neo-tendon (**Fig. 5**). It is of utmost

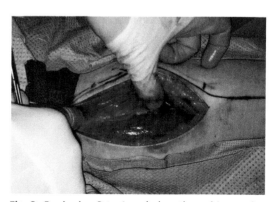

Fig. 3. Beginning 3 to 4 cm below the pubic symphysis, an incision is made between the adductor tubercle and the medial condyle of the femur, 10 to 15 cm in length. The incision is carried down to the muscular fascia, and the gracilis muscle is identified. (*Courtesy of* B. Azizzadeh MD, Beverly Hills, CA.)

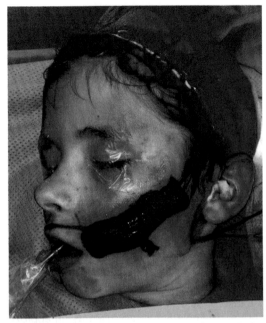

Fig. 4. Approximate desired size of the flap and ultimate configuration of the nerve/vessels. (*Courtesy of* B. Azizzadeh MD, Beverly Hills, CA.)

importance to make sure that the neurovascular bundle is not separated from the underbelly of the muscle during the harvest (**Fig. 6**). The obturator nerve and vessels are dissected to achieve maximal length. The vessels are taken down only after the face has been fully dissected and vessels identified. The leg incision is then closed in the standard fashion after the take-down of the vessels.

On the paralytic side, a modified Blair incision is made and a deep subcutaneous flap is elevated. The SMAS is incised at the anterior border of the parotid gland and a sub-SMAS flap is raised to the level of the oral commissure/nasolabial fold.

Buccal fat is removed as needed to reduce facial bulk in anticipation of the added bulk of the flap. The facial artery and vein are identified and prepared for revascularization. Four to 6 anchoring O-Vicryl sutures are placed in the oral commissure, melolabial and nasolabial folds to be used for the inset of the gracilis flap. With each suture placement, tension is placed on the suture to mimic contraction of the muscle, ensuring appropriate restoration of the oral commissure and nasolabial fold. The sutures are then loosely secured to the gracilis muscle. Using a trochar, the obturator nerve from the gracilis muscle is then passed deep to the sutures into the gingivobuccal sulcus where the distal end of the sural nerve graft was previously placed, and the neurorrhaphy is performed (**Figs. 7** and **8**). The gracilis muscle is subsequently parachuted into the wound, and the loose sutures are firmly tied at the oral commissure and nasolabial fold (**Fig. 9**). The other end of the muscle is attached to the temporoparietal fascia just above the zygoma. The angle of inset is critical to a favorable outcome in restoration of the correct smile angle (**Fig. 10**). At conclusion of the inset, there should be a slight overexaggeration to the nasolabial fold and oral commissure, as some degree of relaxation will occur postoperatively (**Fig. 11**).

The arterial anastomosis is performed using 9-0 nylon suture under the operating microscope, and the venous anastomosis is performed using a coupling device (**Fig. 12**). The location of the arterial anastomosis is marked to allow for postoperative monitoring. Drains are placed and the incision is closed in a layered fashion.

Postoperative Care/Rehabilitation

At conclusion of the procedure, a rectal aspirin is administered. Patients are admitted to the facility

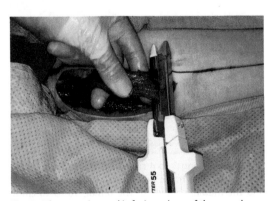

Fig. 5. The superior and inferior edges of the muscle are transected using a GIA stapler creating a neo-tendon. (*Courtesy of* B. Azizzadeh MD, Beverly Hills, CA.)

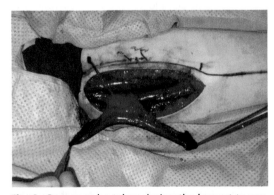

Fig. 6. Care must be taken during the harvest to protect the neurovascular bundle, which lies on the underbelly of the muscle. (*Courtesy of* B. Azizzadeh MD, Beverly Hills, CA.)

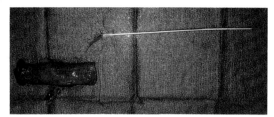

Fig. 7. Using a trochar, the obturator nerve from the gracilis muscle is then passed deep to the sutures into the gingivobuccal sulcus where the distal end of the sural nerve graft was previously placed. (*Courtesy of* B. Azizzadeh MD, Beverly Hills, CA.)

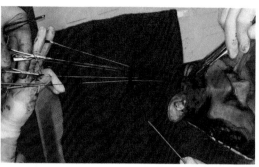

Fig. 9. Four to 6 anchoring O-Vicryl sutures are placed in the oral commissure, and melolabial and nasolabial folds that are used for the inset of the gracilis flap. With each suture placement, tension is placed on the suture to mimic contraction of the muscle, ensuring appropriate restoration of the oral commissure and nasolabial fold. The gracilis muscle is subsequently parachuted into the wound, and the loose sutures are firmly tied at the oral commissure and nasolabial fold. (*Courtesy of* B. Azizzadeh MD, Beverly Hills, CA.)

overnight for observation and hourly Doppler checks. The senior author (BA) has begun performing these operations at an ambulatory surgery center with successful outcomes, the results of which will be published shortly. The patients receive antibiotics, appropriate analgesia, and daily aspirin (81 mg), and are typically discharged the following day to an aftercare facility with the drains in place, to be removed at their first follow-up appointment.

The first muscle contractions typically begin approximately 4 to 6 months postoperatively. Neuromuscular retraining is initiated once patients have started seeing gracilis movement.

OUTCOMES/COMPLICATIONS

The success of the gracilis free muscle transfer in smile restoration has been widely reported.[27,43–45] Several of the senior author's results are demonstrated (**Figs. 13–15**). In the senior author's practice, patients typically begin to experience contractions of the muscle 4 to 6 months after the operation, with strength of contraction gradually

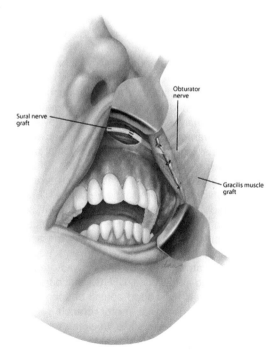

Fig. 8. Illustration of the sural CFNG to the obturator nerve of the gracilis flap. (*Courtesy of* B. Azizzadeh MD, Beverly Hills, CA.)

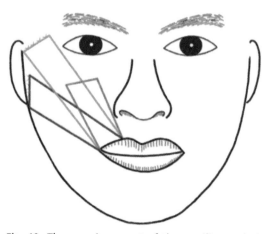

Fig. 10. The superior aspect of the gracilis muscle is sutured to the temporoparietal fascia just above the zygoma. The angle of the inset is critical to restoration of the correct smile angle. (*From* Chuang DC, Lu JC, Anesti K. One-stage procedure using spinal accessory nerve (XI)–innervated free muscle for facial paralysis reconstruction. Plast Reconstr Surg 2013;132(1):128e; with permission.)

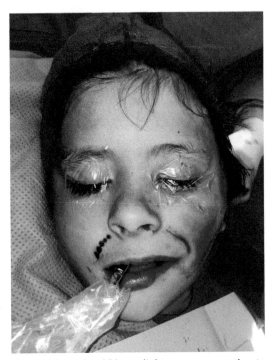

Fig. 11. There should be a slight overexaggeration to the nasolabial fold and oral commissure, as relaxation will occur postoperatively.

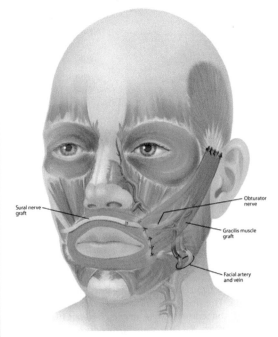

Sural nerve graft

Obturator nerve

Gracilis muscle graft

Facial artery and vein

Fig. 12. Configuration of the vascular anastomosis to the facial artery and vein and completed inset of the flap. (*Courtesy of* B. Azizzadeh MD, Beverly Hills, CA.)

increasing over the course of 12 to 24 months. Facial swelling typically takes 12 months to resolve. Clinical experience has demonstrated that the most common adverse outcomes include lateralization of the nasolabial fold and excessive bulk of the gracilis flap. Experientially, 10% to 20% of patients require a third procedure for repositioning of the nasolabial fold or flap debulking. Others have reported higher rates of need for revision, with some authors proposing a planned third stage.[46]

Overall, flap failure rates due to thrombosis or failure to generate movement are low, with some studies reporting no failures, whereas others have reported rates as high as 9%.[43,47] Other potential procedural complications include damage to the unaffected facial nerve or decreased strength of smile. As with any facial procedure, there is a risk of hematoma.

Of course, all patients will expect to have numbness on the lateral aspect of the foot from sural nerve harvest. There is also a risk of foot drop as a result of accidental damage to the deep peroneal nerve during graft harvest, although this has not been encountered in our experience. Infection rates have been studied by Lee and colleagues,[48] who demonstrated 6 infections in a total of 107 patients undergoing gracilis free tissue transfer. Interestingly, all of these patients were on clindamycin or clindamycin combined with an additional antibiotic. None of the patients with postoperative infections were given ampicillin/sulbactam, suggesting a possible benefit with the use of this antibiotic.

Bhama and colleagues[43] at Massachusetts Eye and Ear Infirmary recently released the results of 154 gracilis free tissue transfers with various donor nerves performed over the past 10 years. To objectively analyze smile function, they developed a new software tool (FaCE-Gram) that uses a number of facial landmarks to evaluate facial movement. They report a 9% flap failure rate. Of those who had a viable flap, 52% used the ipsilateral motor branch of the trigeminal nerve, and 41% were innervated by a CFNG. They found that smile excursion of the paretic side was significantly greater in patients who underwent masseteric innervation, but, likely more relevant, was the finding that smile length symmetry was greater in patients who received a CFNG. Of course, the CFNG also has the added benefit of spontaneity, whereas the trigeminal motor branch required bite action to generate smile. In a later report, the same group also reported a significant improvement in quality of life following gracilis muscle transfer, as determined by a facial disability index.[44]

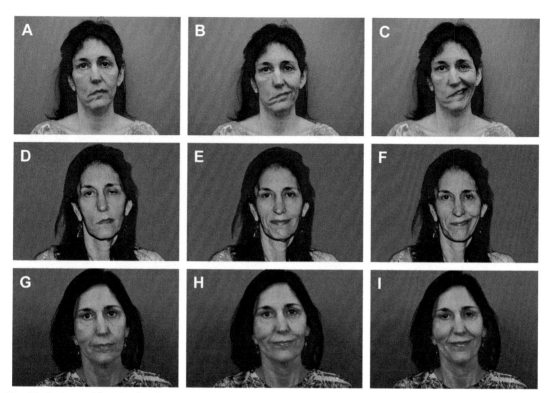

Fig. 13. Patient with right facial paralysis due to an acoustic neuroma. Represented are photographs of the patient at rest, soft smile, and full smile preoperatively (*A–C*), following stage 1 facial nerve to masseteric nerve cranial nerve substitution and CFNG (*D–F*), and after second stage gracilis free flap (*G–I*). (*Courtesy of* B. Azizzadeh MD, Beverly Hills, CA.)

Terzis and Noah[45] also reviewed the results of 100 patients who underwent free muscle transfer at a single institution; 63 patients underwent gracilis muscle transfer, and the remaining majority underwent pectoralis minor transfer. Of the 63 patients who were reanimated with a gracilis free flap, only 1 flap failed to function. The mean time to first contraction was 22.4 ± 9.7 weeks. Restoration of facial function was also assessed on a scale of 1 to 5, with 1 corresponding to poor function and 5 signifying excellent function. The patients treated with a gracilis flap improved by an average of 1.5 points, corresponding to a moderate or greater facial function. Need for revision among the entire cohort was not separated by type of flap used, but of all free muscle transfers, 26% required a subsequent debulking procedure, and 22% required a mini-temporalis transfer to the oral commissure.

In a later report by the same group, long-term outcomes were assessed in 24 patients with at least 5 years of follow-up.[36] They noted one case of flap failure due to thrombosis and another due to failure to function. One patient developed a temporary lower leg paresthesia. All 24 of their patients underwent a third revision surgery. They also noted a continued improvement with time, as compared with their "early" (2-year postoperative) result.

Fig. 14. Patient with developmental right facial nerve paralysis. (*A*) Preoperative smile, and (*B*) 1 year after CFNG and gracilis free flap. The first and second stages were separated by a period of 9 months. (*Courtesy of* B. Azizzadeh MD, Beverly Hills, CA.)

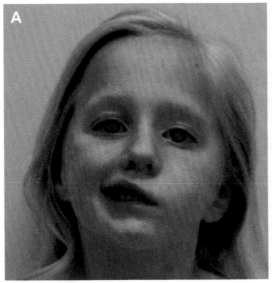
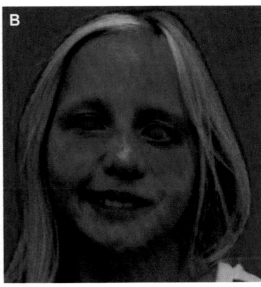

Fig. 15. Preoperative (*A*) and 2 years postoperative photographs (*B*) of a patient with a congenital benign tumor of the posterior cranial fossa and cerebellum. The tumor was excised, resulting in a complete left facial nerve paralysis. She underwent CFNG and gracilis free flap. Her first and second stages were separated by 18 months. She did require a revision procedure to reduce flap bulk. (*Courtesy of* B. Azizzadeh MD, Beverly Hills, CA.).

SUMMARY

Facial paralysis is a disfiguring and life-altering condition with emotional and social implications. For patients with complete or severe unilateral paralysis, dynamic facial reanimation with free muscle transfer has been shown to greatly improve smile symmetry. The gracilis free flap is a very efficacious method of emotive, spontaneous facial expression restoration. A 2-stage procedure with a CFNG is the ideal mode of smile restoration, allowing for spontaneity in expression, which is critical to social interaction not only in smile but also in the ability to demonstrate emotion in conversation. Masseteric nerve is an excellent alternative donor nerve. Dual innervation studies are underway to determine potential benefits.

REFERENCES

1. Coulson SE, O'Dwyer NJ, Adams RD, et al. Expression of emotion and quality of life after facial nerve paralysis. Otology Neurotology 2004;25(6): 1014–9.
2. Sinno H, Thibaudeau S, Izadpanah A, et al. Utility outcome scores for unilateral facial paralysis. Ann Plast Surg 2012;69(4):435–8.
3. Pickrell KL, Broadbent TR, Masters FW, et al. Construction of a rectal sphincter and restoration of anal continence by transplanting the gracilis muscle; a report of four cases in children. Ann Surg 1952;135(6):853–62.
4. Harii K, Ohmori K, Sekiguchi J. The free musculocutaneous flap. Plast Reconstr Surg 1976;57(3): 294–303.
5. Harii K, Ohmori K, Torii S. Free gracilis muscle transplantation, with microneurovascular ansatomoses for the treatment of facial paralysis: a preliminary report. Plast Reconstr Surg 1976;57(2): 133–43.
6. The use of neuromuscular free autografts with microneural anastomosis to restore elevation to the paralysed angle of the mouth in cases of unilateral facial paralysis. Chirurgia Plast 1976;3(3):165–74.
7. O'Brien BM, Pederson WC, Khazanchi R, et al. Results of management of facial palsy with microvascular free-muscle transfer. Plast Reconstr Surg 1990;86(1):12–22.
8. Harrison DH. The pectoralis minor vascularized muscle graft for the treatment of unilateral facial palsy. Plast Reconstr Surg 1985;75(2):206–13.
9. Whitney TM, Buncke HJ, Alpert BS, et al. The serratus anterior free-muscle flap: experience with 100 consecutive cases. Plast Reconstr Surg 1990; 86(3):481–90.
10. Dellon AL, Mackinnon SE. Segmentally innervated latissimus dorsi muscle. Microsurgical transfer for facial reanimation. J Reconstr Microsurgery 1985; 2(1):7–12.
11. Harii K, Asato H, Yoshimura K, et al. One-stage transfer of the latissimus dorsi muscle for

reanimation of a paralyzed face: a new alternative. Plast Reconstr Surg 1998;102(4):941–51.

12. Hata Y, Yano K, Matsuka K, et al. Treatment of chronic facial palsy by transplantation of the neuro-vascularized free rectus abdominis muscle. Plast Reconstr Surg 1990;86(6):1178–87.

13. Koshima I, Moriguchi T, Soeda S, et al. Free rectus femoris muscle transfer for one-stage reconstruction of established facial paralysis. Plast Reconstr Surg 1994;94(3):421–30.

14. Harrison DH, Grobbelaar AO. Pectoralis minor muscle transfer for unilateral facial palsy reanimation: an experience of 35 years and 637 cases. J Plast Reconstr Aesthet Surg 2012;65(7):845–50.

15. Takushima A, Harii K, Asato H, et al. One-stage reconstruction of facial paralysis associated with skin/soft tissue defects using latissimus dorsi compound flap. J Plast Reconstr Aesthet Surg 2006; 59(5):465–73.

16. Takushima A, Harii K, Asato H, et al. Fifteen-year survey of one-stage latissimus dorsi muscle transfer for treatment of longstanding facial paralysis. J Plast Reconstr Aesthet Surg 2013;66(1):29–36.

17. Alam DS, Haffey T, Vakharia K, et al. Sternohyoid flap for facial reanimation: a comprehensive preclinical evaluation of a novel technique. JAMA Facial Plast Surg 2013;15(4):305–13.

18. Juricic M, Vaysse PH, Guitard J, et al. Anatomic basis for use of a gracilis muscle flap. Surg Radiologic Anat 1993;15(3):163–8.

19. Magden O, Tayfur V, Edizer M, et al. Anatomy of gracilis muscle flap. J Craniofac Surg 2010;21(6): 1948–50.

20. Papadopoulos O, Georgiou P, Christopoulos A, et al. The gracilis flap revisited. Eur J Plast Surg 2000; 23(8):413–8.

21. Updhyaya D, Khanna V, Bhattacharya S, et al. The transversely split gracilis twin free flaps. Indian J Plast Surg 2010;43(2):173–6.

22. Smith JW. A new technique of facial reanimation. In: Hueston JT, editor. Transactions of the 5th international congress of plastic surgery. London: Butterworths; 1971. p. 83.

23. Scaramella L. L'anastomosi tra I due nervi facciali. Arch Otolaryngol 1971;82:209.

24. Scaramella LF. Cross-face facial nerve anastomosis: historical notes. Ear Nose Throat J 1996;123(6): 1697–703.

25. Kumar PA, Hassan KM. Cross-face nerve graft with free-muscle transfer for reanimation of the paralyzed face: a comparative study of the single-stage and two-stage procedures. Plast Reconstr Surg 2002; 109(2):451–62.

26. Hontanilla B, Marre D, Cabello Á. Facial reanimation with gracilis muscle transfer neurotized to cross-facial nerve graft versus masseteric nerve: a comparative study using the FACIAL CLIMA evaluating system. Plast Reconstr Surg 2013; 131(6):1241–52.

27. Bae YC, Zuker RM, Manktelow RT, et al. A comparison of commissure excursion following gracilis muscle transplantation for facial paralysis using a cross-face nerve graft versus the motor nerve to the masseter nerve. Plast Reconstr Surg 2006;117(7):2407–13.

28. Manktelow RT, Tomat LR, Zuker RM, et al. Smile reconstruction in adults with free muscle transfer innervated by the masseter motor nerve: effectiveness and cerebral adaptation. Plast Reconstr Surg 2006;118(4):885–99.

29. Gousheh J, Arasteh E. Treatment of facial paralysis: dynamic reanimation of spontaneous facial expression—apropos of 655 patients. Plast Reconstr Surg 2011;128(6):693e–703e.

30. McCabe BF. Facial nerve grafting. Plast Reconstr Surg 1970;45(1):70–5.

31. Barrs DM. Facial nerve trauma: optimal timing for repair. Laryngoscope 1991;101(8):835–48.

32. Guntinas-Lichius O. The facial nerve in the presence of head and neck neoplasm: assessment and outcome after surgical management. Curr Opin Otolaryngol Head Neck Surg 2004;12(2): 133–41.

33. Anastomosis of masseteric nerve to lower division of facial nerve for correction of lower facial paralysis, preliminary report. Plast Reconstr Surg 1978;61(3): 330–4.

34. Hypoglossal-facial nerve anastomosis for reinnervation of the paralyzed face. Plast Reconstr Surg 1979; 63(1):63–72.

35. Baker D. Hypoglossal facial nerve anastomosis indications and limitations. Proceedings Fifth International Symposium facial nerve. New York: Masson Publ; 1985. p. 526–9.

36. Terzis JK, Tzafetta K. The "babysitter" procedure: minihypoglossal to facial nerve transfer and cross-facial nerve grafting. Plast Reconstr Surg 2009; 123(3):865–76.

37. Terzis JK. "Babysitters." An exciting new concept in facial reanimation. In: Proceedings of the 6th International Symposium on the facial nerve, Rio de Janiero, Brazil, October 2–5, 1988. Amsterdam (The Netherlands); Berkeley (CA); Milano (Italy): Kugler & Ghedini; 1990. p. 525.

38. Faria JC, Scopel GP, Ferreira MC. Facial reanimation with masseteric nerve: babysitter or permanent procedure? Preliminary results. Ann Plast Surg 2010; 64(1):31–4.

39. Hoffmann D. Bilateral facial paralysis. Otology Neurotology 2002;23:S32.

40. Hadlock TA, Cheney ML. Single-incision endoscopic sural nerve harvest for cross face nerve grafting. J Reconstr Microsurg 2008;24(7): 519–23.

41. Peng GL, Azizzadeh B. Cross-facial nerve grafting for facial reanimation. Facial Plast Surg 2015;31(2): 128–33.

42. Braam MJ, Nicolai JP. Axonal regeneration rate through cross-face nerve grafts. Microsurgery 1993;19(9):589–91.

43. Bhama PK, Weinberg JS, Lindsay RW, et al. Objective outcomes analysis following microvascular gracilis transfer for facial reanimation. JAMA Facial Plast Surg 2014;16(2):85–92.

44. Lindsay RW, Bhama P, Hadlock TA. Quality-of-life improvement after free gracilis muscle transfer for smile restoration in patients with facial paralysis. JAMA Facial Plast Surg 2014;16(6): 419–24.

45. Terzis JK, Noah ME. Analysis of 100 cases of free-muscle transplantation for facial paralysis. Int Inst Reconstr Microsurgery 1996;99(7):1905–21.

46. Chuang DC. Technique evolution for facial paralysis reconstruction using functioning free muscle transplantation—experience of Chang Gung Memorial Hospital. Clin Plast Surg 2002;29(4):449–59.

47. Ferreira MC, Marques de Faria JC. Result of microvascular gracilis transplantation for facial paralysis–personal series. Clin Plast Surg 2002;29(4): 515–22.

48. Lee LN, Susarla SM, Henstrom DK, et al. Surgical site infections after gracilis free flap reconstruction for facial paralysis. Otolaryngol Head Neck Surg 2012;147(2):245–8.

The Sternohyoid Flap for Facial Reanimation

Daniel S. Alam, MD

KEYWORDS

- Facial paralysis • Free flap • Facial reanimation • Microvascular • Gracilis • Sternohyoid

KEY POINTS

- The sternohyoid muscle can be harvested as a free flap for microvascular transfer.
- The sternohyoid offers comparatively better anatomic size match to the zygomaticus major muscle compared with the gracilis.
- The sternohyoid has a better fiber type match to the zygomaticus major based on ATPase staining.
- Early clinical outcomes are promising, but significant further study and long-term outcomes must be evaluated before this flap can supplant the gracilis as the gold standard for neuromuscular free flap based facial reanimation.

INTRODUCTION

The rehabilitation facial nerve paralysis associated with nerve transection is ideally accomplished through neuromuscular reanimation of the face. When possible, the best case scenario is reestablishing a neural connection between the native facial nerve branch and its specific facial musculature target at a distal location in the nerve that would restore to the closest approximation normal facial function. Unfortunately this ideal situation is rarely encountered in the clinical setting. In most cases, nerve transection or resection occurs proximal to the pes anserinus, which in turn inherently predisposes recovery to synkinesis. Even this option becomes unavailable in long-standing cases of paralysis. Beyond 18 to 24 months after injury, the motor endplates of the denervated muscles irreversibly atrophy. In this situation, a neuromuscular transfer incorporating both a new neural input source and muscular mechanism is necessary. The 2 most commonly used options in these circumstances are local transfer of the temporalis tendon in an orthodromic fashion or free muscle transfer utilizing the gracilis muscle. These 2 options are discussed in other articles within this issue.

Of the free tissue transfer options, the most commonly used and widely accepted is the gracilis flap. This is at present considered the gold standard for microvascular flaps used in reanimation procedures. In an optimal outcome, this technique allows the rehabilitation of a spontaneous smile. This muscle has become the mainstay of free tissue facial reanimation. It is used widely in pediatric and adult indications with relatively good outcomes and results.[1–3] The ease of harvest and reliability of the flap have made it an excellent option in patients with long-standing paralysis.

The use of this flap is not, however, without its limitations. There are anatomic parameters of the gracilis that can make the results suboptimal. The most frequently cited concern is the bulk of the flap, especially in relation to the temporal region and the zygoma. The skin envelope and soft tissue overlying the zygoma in adults are generally less than 8 mm thick. Draping a free muscle flap over this convex bony landmark often creates a visible facial deformity.[4] This is less than ideal given the purpose of facial nerve rehabilitation and reanimation is to reduce physical deformity. The flap works well in children and young adults with ample facial volume, but when used in older

The Queen's Head and Neck Institute, John A Burns School of Medicine, University of Hawaii, 130 Punchbowl Street, Honolulu, HI 96813, USA
E-mail address: dan.alam@hotmail.com

Facial Plast Surg Clin N Am 24 (2016) 61–69
http://dx.doi.org/10.1016/j.fsc.2015.09.005
1064-7406/16/$ – see front matter © 2016 Elsevier Inc. All rights reserved.

facialplastic.theclinics.com

patients who are usually affected by parotid malignancy and who usually have concurrent weight loss and facial atrophy, the flap is difficult to camouflage.

Many authors have reported successful volume reduction of the harvested gracilis flap as a modification to reduce this problem.[5] Even with such pre-emptive measures, the muscle bulk is significantly larger than the zygomaticus major/minor that the gracilis is intended to functionally replace. Not surprisingly, the flap is noted to be more favorable aesthetically in younger patients, in whom the facial soft tissue envelope is proportionately thicker and more robust.

The numerous modifications of the gracilis reported in the literature highlight the historical reality that this flap was not originally designed and reported as a means to rehabilitate facial nerve paralysis. Initial reports in the literature and the widespread use of this flap were for indications in the peripheral extremities (eg, wound coverage).[6–8] Over time, the flap has been regarded as a well-established muscle flap with a reliable pedicle and nerve input that could be harvested with ease. This clinical history and reliability led to its eventual use in the face, but the choice of this muscle for this particular indication was not based on a directed search for the ideal muscle to replace facial musculature.

There are other characteristics of the gracilis flap that are less than ideal. When considering a number of parameters, including muscle size, length contraction/ratio, intrinsic type 1/type 2 fiber ratios (although these can shift to some extent with reinnervation in certain muscle transfers), the muscle is quite distinct from the Zygomaticus major.[9]

An anatomic comparison of the 2 muscles is shown in **Fig. 1**. The images illustrate an obvious difference in the size of the muscles. The average length of the gracilis muscle in an adult man is 41 cm, and only a small portion of the muscle is harvested in a facial reanimation procedure. The length/contraction ratio of the muscle for the lengths harvested for facial reanimation is therefore unfavorable in contrast to that seen in the zygomaticus major, which only averages 5 cm in length and can have discursion over 2 cm in some cases.

Another potential difference is in muscle physiology. A comparison of fast twitch type II muscle fiber activity of the gracilis to the zygomaticus major shows significant differences between these muscles. The author's findings are shown in **Fig. 2**, and they corroborate the accepted literature. This is not unexpected when one considers the purpose of these muscles and their function within their native location. The gracilis is a muscle

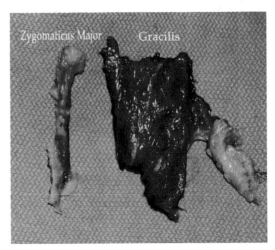

Fig. 1. An equivalent length of zygomaticus major (*left*) and harvested gracilis flap (*right*) for comparison of size and volume.

that is involved in chronic low-grade contraction associated with maintaining balance and stability of the torso. The zygomaticus major, in contrast, is involved in rapid facial expression and has almost the highest ratio of fast twitch fibers of any muscle in the body just behind the orbicularis oculi.

Because muscle fiber type is thought to be determined by the neural innervation source, this may not represent a clinical problem, but the limited data available on gracilis flaps suggest this transformation is not seen clinically.[10,11]

This led the author and colleagues to a directed need-based search for an alternative to the gracilis as a potential free flap for facial reanimation. Ideally, this flap would have several characteristics:

1. Reliable and nonessential vascular pedicle
2. Motor nerve input with a reliable nerve (nonessential function, appropriate length, diameter, branching)
3. Fast twitch muscle fibers with a rapid and brisk contraction profile or clinical evidence of fiber type transition with reinnervation
4. Shorter length from origin to insertion and a superior length/contraction ratio
5. Rigid or semirigid origin/insertion point for better fixation
6. Smaller muscle mass and size (**Fig. 3**)

Using these criteria, the author and colleagues hypothesized the sternohyoid muscle potentially could be an ideal replacement. The vascular supply of the strap muscles had been previously shown as potentially reliable for use as a pedicled

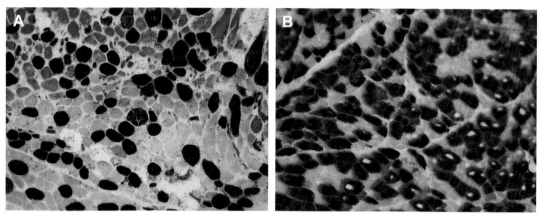

Fig. 2. High power microscopic views of ATPase staining at pH 4.6. Type I fibers stain dark with this reagent and the fast twitch Type II fibers are light. Panel (*A*) shows the zygomaticus major; panel (*B*) shows the gracilis.

flap,[12] but its potential use as a free flap had not been reported.

The findings of a preclinical, cadaver-based study that described this novel flap were reported in *The Archives of Facial Plastic Surgery*. Details of the operative technique and a comprehensive description of the flap are provided from that study. Specific diagrams are reprinted here with permission.

The conclusion of this work documented that the sternohyoid muscle could reliably be harvested as a free flap with a pedicle based on the superior thyroid vessel. A representative angiogram is shown in **Fig. 4**. The flap has a pedicle

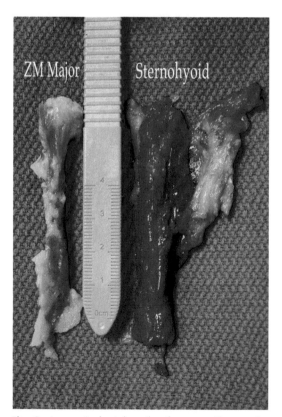

Fig. 3. An equivalent length of zygomaticus major (*left*) and harvested sternohyoid flap (*right*) for comparison of size and volume.

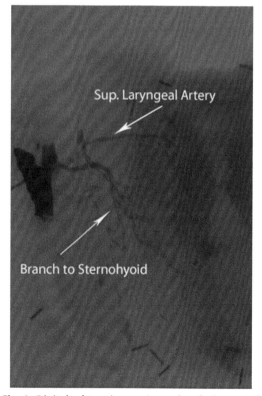

Fig. 4. Digital subtraction angiography of a harvested sternohyoid flap. The injection study shows the perfusion of the muscle through the descending branch as well as some superior perfusion through the superior laryngeal branch.

length of over 5 cm and a reliable long motor nerve in the ansa branches.

SURGICAL TECHNIQUE

The surgical steps of the harvest are shown in **Figs. 5–8**.

A hemiapron incision is made centered in a neck crease between the hyoid and the sternum just superior to the placement of the typical incision for a thyroidectomy. Subplatysmal flaps are then elevated to expose the underlying strap muscles and the sternocleidomastoid muscle (SCM). The SCM is retracted laterally to expose the great vessels and identify the ansa cervicalis. This is dissected from its origin at the hypoglossal nerve to point of innervation of the sternohyoid (SH) approximately 2 cm above the sternum. The omohyoid is divided to facilitate the completion of this dissection (see **Fig. 5**)

The external carotid artery is dissected to identify the origin of the superior thyroid artery (STA). The STA is dissected distally, with care taken to identify and preserve the accompanying pedicle vein (see **Fig. 6**).

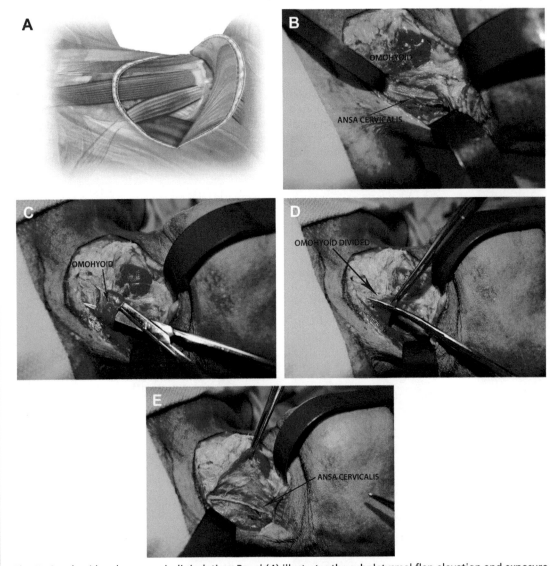

Fig. 5. Omohyoid and ansa cervicalis isolation. Panel (*A*) illustrates the subplatysmal flap elevation and exposure. Panel (*B*) shows retraction of the omohyoid and exposure of the ansa on the superficial surface of the internal jugular vein. Panel (*C*) shows isolation of the omohyoid, which is in turn, divided in panel (*D*). Panel (*E*) reveals the ansa fully exposed. ([*A*] *From* Alam DS, Haffey T, Vakharia K, et al. Sternohyoid flap for facial reanimation: a comprehensive preclinical evaluation of a novel technique. JAMA Facial Plast Surg 2013;15(4):305–13; with permission.)

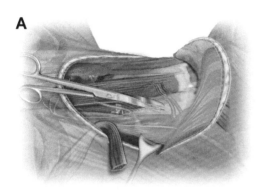
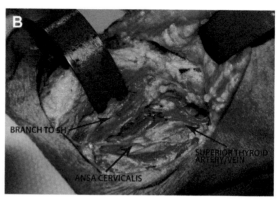

Fig. 6. Vascular pedicle dissection. Panel (*A*) illustrates the great vessel dissection to isolate the superior thyroid artery pedicle. Panel (*B*) shows the completed pedicle dissection with the branch to the sternohyoid noted on the image. Distal ligation at the superior pole of the thyroid completes this dissection. ([*A*] *From* Alam DS, Haffey T, Vakharia K, et al. Sternohyoid flap for facial reanimation: a comprehensive preclinical evaluation of a novel technique. JAMA Facial Plast Surg 2013;15(4):305–13; with permission.)

The STA is then suture ligated distal to the medial branches to the sternohyoid at the superior pole of the ipsilateral thyroid gland lobe.

A second potential venous outflow through the middle thyroid vein may be isolated at this point.

The proximal vein pedicle is then dissected to draining vein with a luminal diameter of 2 to 3 mm. This is most often seen with the ranine veins associated with the hypoglossal nerve, but in some cases directly into the internal jugular.

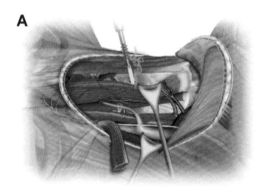
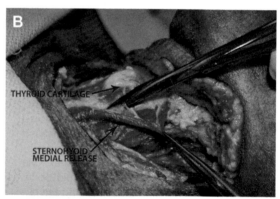
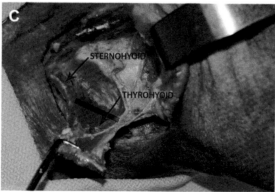

Fig. 7. Medial release of flap. Panel (*A*) illustrates the medal release of the flap in diagrammatic form. Panel (*B*) show separation of the sternohyoid from the thyroid cartilage. Panel (*C*) shows the attachments of the thyrohyoid muscle with the release point noted with the shaded rectangle. The sternothyroid also must be released. ([*A*] *From* Alam DS, Haffey T, Vakharia K, et al. Sternohyoid flap for facial reanimation: a comprehensive preclinical evaluation of a novel technique. JAMA Facial Plast Surg 2013;15(4):305–13; with permission.)

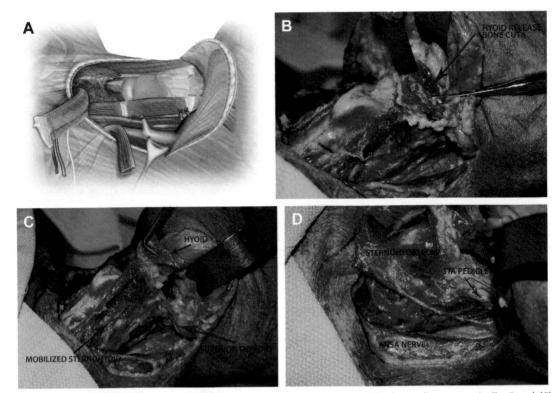

Fig. 8. Hyoid release and flap mobilization: panel (*A*) illustrates the hyoid release diagrammatically. Panel (*B*) shows isolation of the hyoid and planned saw cuts around the central sternohyoid attachment. Panel (*C*) shows the mobilized hyoid/sternohyoid complex. Panel (*D*) shows the entire harvested flap in situ after the inferior sternohyoid release. ([*A*] *From* Alam DS, Haffey T, Vakharia K, et al. Sternohyoid flap for facial reanimation: a comprehensive preclinical evaluation of a novel technique. JAMA Facial Plast Surg 2013;15(4):305–13; with permission.)

The SH is reflected posterolaterally as the thyrohyoid and sternothyroid attachments are released from the thyroid cartilage (see **Fig. 7**).

The superior release is performed next via isolation of the anterior face of the hyoid bone. The suprahyoid muscles are released and the hyoid cut medial and lateral to the attachment to the ipsilateral sternohyoid. Care is taken to avoid injury to the underlying hypoglossal nerve (see **Fig. 8**).

Finally, the inferior muscle cut is made below the level where the ansa fibers innervate the muscle body.

The harvested flap is shown in **Fig. 9**.

The inset technique is shown is **Fig. 10**. The muscle is anchored with rigid fixation of the superior hyoid attachment to the superior and inner surface of the zygoma with a 1.0 mm microplate. This allows rigid fixation with minimal if any temporal fossa distortion. The pedicle is anastomosed to the superficial temporal artery and the superficial and/or deep temporal vein. Alternatively, the pedicle length allows the use of the facial vessels (artery, vein), but this would have an expected size mismatch. The distal muscle is suture fixed at the modiolus and can be divided to attach around the commissure, as is often done with the gracilis.

One unique advantage is the graft length of the recipient nerve that can easily be transferred in a single stage across the upper lip in a subcutaneous plane to the contralateral facial nerve

Fig. 9. Example of the harvested flap.

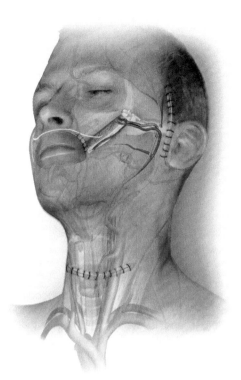

Fig. 10. Inset characteristics for use in facial reanimation. (*From* Alam DS, Haffey T, Vakharia K, et al. Sternohyoid flap for facial reanimation: a comprehensive preclinical evaluation of a novel technique. JAMA Facial Plast Surg 2013;15(4):305–13; with permission.)

due to its long average length. This is shown in **Fig. 11**.

FLAP CHARACTERISTICS

Angiography of the pedicle revealed brisk perfusion of the entire muscle, as well as a venous phase to the superior thyroid vein. A lengthy

vascular pedicle was identified in all specimens, with an average pedicle length of 5.5 cm.

The fiber type match was assessed with ATPase staining shown in **Fig. 12**. The fast twitch brisk contraction fibers seen in the native Zygomaticus major are much more analogous to those seen in the sternohyoid compared with the gracilis. Based their findings, the author and colleagues felt this flap had significant potential advantages over the gracilis. The ansa nerve is 10.7 cm in average length. The author's comprehensive evaluation of the harvest, clinical parameters, and preclinical evaluation of the inset for use in facial reanimation was the first report of the use of the sternohyoid muscle as a potential new free flap.

The ultimate measure of the success or failure of a particular novel approach is clinical success in actual patients. A clinical trial of the procedure has been undertaken, and to date 5 patients have been recruited into the study. The detailed outcomes and results of this study remain unpublished of the timing of this publication, as the time frame to reinnervation and functional outcomes has not been met for many of the patients in the trial. Preliminary results have been promising based on early observations, but detailed presentation of this data is beyond the scope of this report.

The clinical outcome of the first patient 6 months postoperatively is shown in **Fig. 13**. This patient had a history of a parotid malignancy and resection of the facial nerve, with a 3-year interval to reanimation. Options for neural rehabilitation using nerve transfer (masseter or hypoglossal facial) were therefore not feasible because of the loss of motor end plates. The patient was given the option of temporalis tendon transfer, a gracilis flap, or the sternohyoid flap for his reanimation. He chose the latter.

Given his advanced age and thin facial soft tissue envelope, camouflage of the gracilis would

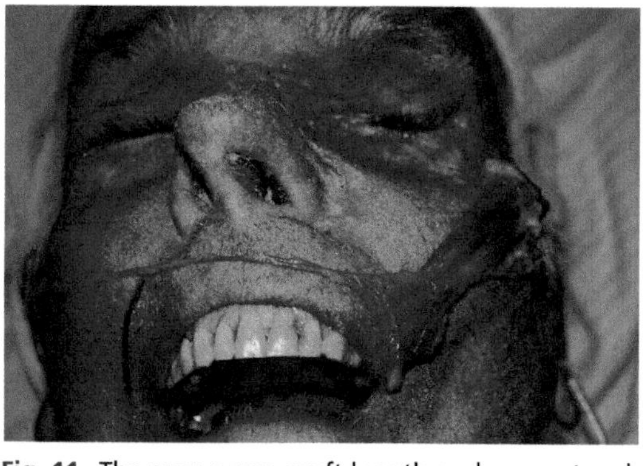

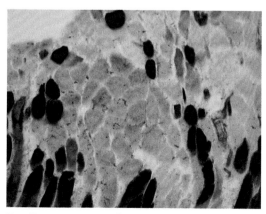

Fig. 11. The ansa nerve graft length and geometry allows for immediate single stage cross facial nerve coaptation.

Fig. 12. ATPase stain of sternohyoid muscle.

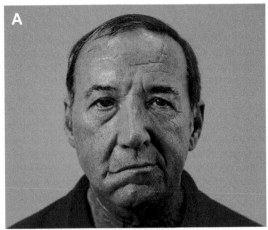 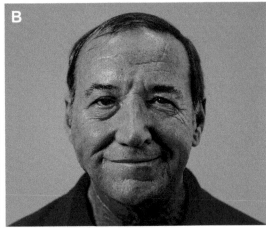

Fig. 13. Panel (*A*) shows patient at rest. Panel (*B*) show patient with attempted smile.

have been challenging in this case. The skin and subcutaneous overlying the zygoma were only 5 mm thick, and the patient had undergone prior radiation treatment to the face and wound bed as adjuvant therapy. His case represented the exact clinical scenario in which traditional neuromuscular free flaps would have been less than ideal, but the potential anatomic advantages of the sternohyoid flap would be favorable.

The patient underwent a sternohyoid flap using an ipsilateral masseter nerve donor. His outcomes highlight the advantages of physical characteristics of the flap that are favorable to its counterparts. There is minimal bulk, and it is well camouflaged even in this thin older patient. The contraction seen is brisk, and the total discursion from rest to full contraction is 22 mm, making it is equal to that seen of a full smile on his normal side. In their assessment of this result, the author and colleagues believe this is because of the favorable length to contraction/ratio of the sternohyoid muscle. Even though the total length of the sternohyoid is only 8-10 cm, the muscle can contract almost 30% with potential discursions of over 2-3 cm.

In their hands, especially when considering the older patient population found in malignant etiologies, the author and colleagues were not able to achieve this type of result with the gracilis or any other neuromuscular free flap alternatives. Those flaps were bulky and noticeable despite the author's efforts at volumetric size reduction. The end result was often trading 1 physical deformity (akinesis) for another (bulky disfiguration). The clinical significance of this observation bears critical importance to the potential widespread clinical application of this technique. Numerically, the older iatrogenically paralyzed patient population

is much more common than the childhood presentation of facial paralysis that is often managed by free flaps, and it is this older group that often goes undertreated. These patients are often treated by less invasive or quicker approaches. Many of these techniques, including static slings and temporalis tendon transfer, are discussed separately in this issue. They clearly have their merits and are utilized frequently by this author as well. Having said that, it should be noted, that while these are acceptable clinical alternatives and they will undoubtedly improve patient quality of life, the author not found them capable of achieving type of results seen with the sternohyoid flap.

As a caveat to the reader, the interpretation of these findings must be guarded. At this stage, the outcome is simply a case report, and the complete evaluation of the flap remains a study in progress. Once the study is closed, and the long-term data are assessed, the author and colleagues can provide a more definitive conclusion, as well as more concrete practice recommendations. Until that point, this is simply a discussion of a novel technique with promise.

REFERENCES

1. Manktelow RT, Tomat LR, Zuker RM, et al. Smile reconstruction in adults with free muscle transfer innervated by the masseter motor nerve: effectiveness and cerebral adaptation. Plast Reconstr Surg 2006;118(4):885–99.
2. Hadlock TA, Malo JS, Cheney ML, et al. Free gracilis transfer for smile in children: the Massachusetts Eye and Ear Infirmary experience in excursion and quality-of-life changes. Arch Facial Plast Surg 2011;13(3):190–4.

3. Terzis JK, Tzafetta K. Babysitter procedure with concomitant muscle transfer in facial paralysis. Plast Reconstr Surg 2009;124(4):1142–56.
4. Frey M, Michaelidou M, Tzou CH, et al. Three-dimensional video analysis of the paralyzed face reanimated by cross-face nerve grafting and free gracilis muscle transplantation: quantification of the functional outcome. Plast Reconstr Surg 2008; 122(6):1709–22.
5. Zuker RM, Goldberg CS, Manktelow RT. Facial animation in children with Möbius syndrome after segmental gracilis muscle transplant. Plast Reconstr Surg 2000;106(1):1–8 [discussion: 9].
6. Pu LL. Soft-tissue reconstruction of an open tibial wound in the distal third of the leg: a new treatment algorithm. Ann Plast Surg 2007;58(1):78–83.
7. Haasbeek JF, Zuker RM, Wright JG. Free gracilis muscle transfer for coverage of severe foot deformities. J Pediatr Orthop 1995;15(5):608–12.

8. Soper JT, Rodriguez G, Berchuck A, et al. Long and short gracilis myocutaneous flaps for vulvovaginal reconstruction after radical pelvic surgery: comparison of flap-specific complications. Gynecol Oncol 1995;56(2):271–5.
9. Shimozawa A, Ishizuya-Oka A. Muscle fiber type analysis in the mouse m. digastricus, m. stylohyoideus, m. zygomaticus and m. buccinator. Anat Anz 1987;164(5):355–61.
10. Kauhanen SC, Ylä-Kotola TM, Leivo IV, et al. Long-term adaptation of human microneurovascular muscle flaps to the paralyzed face: an immunohistochemical study. Microsurgery 2006;26(8):557–65.
11. Rhee HS, Hoh JF. Immunohistochemical analysis of the effects of cross-innervation of murine thyroarytenoid and sternohyoid muscles. J Histochem Cytochem 2010;58(12):1057–65.
12. Wang RC, Puig CM, Brown DJ. Strap muscle neurovascular supply. Laryngoscope 1998;108(7):973–6.

Neural Reanimation Advances and New Technologies

Jennifer Kim, MD

KEYWORDS

- Facial reanimation • Nerve substitution • Hypoglossal nerve transfer • Masseteric nerve transfer
- Facial nerve regeneration • Nerve conduit • Facial paralysis treatment

KEY POINTS

- Review of peripheral nerve anatomy, injury, and repair.
- The goal of facial reanimation is to restore facial symmetry and function by primary nerve repair whenever possible, followed by nerve substitution.
- There is an explosion of applicable technology related to biomedical and tissue engineering toward facial reanimation.

 Videos of patients after neural reanimation surgery accompany this article at http://www.facialplastic.theclinics.com/

There is no treatment that can guarantee total recovery and normalization of function following repair of an injured nerve. The poor outcome reflects the complexity of peripheral nerve injuries and the diversity of cellular and biochemical events required to regain function. Facial reanimation has been an area of much research by surgeons, research scientists, biomedical engineers, and tissue engineers due to the devastating impact of facial paralysis aesthetically and functionally. This article focuses on advances in neural reanimation as well as new technologies on the horizon.

This will include discussion of nerve repair, cable grafting, nerve substitution procedures, use of conduits, autografts and allografts, and future directions.

NERVE INJURY

It is important to review the process of nerve injury and repair when considering therapeutic strategies to simultaneously potentiate axonal regeneration, neuronal survival, modulate central reorganization, and inhibit target organ atrophy. The processes of nerve regeneration and target reinnervation are complex, involving physiologic, biochemical, and cellular changes throughout the whole length of the neuron.[1]

From the moment of injury, the distal nerve stump undergoes Wallerian degeneration, while the proximal stump retracts and the Schwann cells activate nearby macrophages to clear the injured axon.[2]

In addition to debris removal, Schwann cells serve several other functions important for recovery from nerve damage. Whereas these cells normally provide axonal myelin to enhance action potential conduction speed, axon transection causes Schwann cells in the distal end of the transected nerve to switch from a myelination phenotype to a growth-supportive one.[3]

The axon sprouts and a growth cone is formed at the tip of each sprout, interacting with activated and proliferating Schwann cells.[4]

Disclosure Statement: The author has nothing to disclose.
Department of Otolaryngology-Head and Neck Surgery, University of Michigan Health System, 1904 TC, 1500 East Medical Center Drive, Ann Arbor, MI 48109, USA
E-mail address: jennkim@med.umich.edu

facialplastic.theclinics.com

Changes also occur to the proximal neuronal cell bodies in dorsal root ganglia with a shift in protein synthesis from a "signaling mode" to a "growing mode" and protein synthesis switches from neurotransmitter-related substances to those required for axonal reconstruction.[5] The gap at the injury site is aligned by Schwann cells coming from the distal stump to form columns of cells called the bands of Bungner.[6] These columns act as a natural "conduit" to guide and help the regenerating axons reach the end organ. Dedifferentiated Schwann cells upregulate the expression of many regeneration-related elements, such as laminin and collagen, which make up the vital extracellular matrix of the nerve.[7] Regeneration involves contact guidance between the growing axon tip and the Schwann cells lining the tube. The regenerated axon must reinnervate the proper target, and the target must retain the ability to accept reinnervation and recover from denervation-related atrophy.[7] Regeneration rate is approximately 1 mm per day; therefore, more proximal injuries lead to longer denervation periods.[8]

Understanding the complex process of regeneration has spurred research in tissue engineering of natural and artificial conduits and the emerging role of cell-based supportive therapies in nerve repair.[9–12]

NERVE ANATOMY

It is also important to understand the structural anatomy of the nerve, which includes mesoneurium, epineurium, perineurium, and endoneurium.[13] The mesoneurium is a connective tissue sheath that suspends the nerve trunk within the soft tissue that contains the segmental blood supply to the nerve. The epineurium is a layer of loose scattered fibroblasts, and adipocytes that defines the nerve trunk and provides mechanical protection. Within the nerve trunk, the perineurium is a multilayered sheath of flattened and densely packed supporting pericytes that surrounds groups of axons, and subdivides the nerve into fascicular bundles. Additionally, the perineurium is the major contributor to nerve tensile strength, serves as a diffusion barrier analogous to the blood-nerve barrier, and contains a latticework for vascular bed. The endoneurium is a loose collagenous matrix within each nerve fascicle that surrounds the individual axons and their Schwann cells (Fig. 1).

The blood supply to the peripheral nerve is a complex vascular plexus fed by radicular vessels in the mesoneurium. Anastomotic connections between epineurial and perineurial plexi occur at

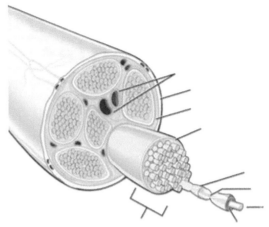

Fig. 1. Schematic presentation of peripheral nerve anatomy. A peripheral nerve is composed of axons of multiple neurons bundled in connective tissue fascicles surrounded by perineurium. Within the nerve, microvasculature runs along the outer layer (epineurium) with a transverse capillary network perfusing the endoneurium. Each fascile itself is composed of endoneurium containing multiple neurons surrounded with myelin produced by Schwann cells. (*From* Siemionow M, Brzezicki G. Current techniques and concepts in peripheral nerve repair. Int Rev Neurobiol 2009;87:143; with permission.)

various levels in the perineurium and eventually arborize into the network of endoneurial capillaries. This vascular plexus is exquisitely sensitive to tension, as animal studies have demonstrated an 80% decrease in blood flow and irreversible ischemic damage with a 15% increase in nerve tension.[14]

Hence, the development of cable grafts and conduits to provide tension-free coaptation and intact vascularity for successful regeneration. It is important to realize and educate the patient that the preinjury facial form and function is never attainable.

NERVE REPAIR

There are 3 surgical reconstruction strategies: (1) direct repair, in which the proximal and distal nerve ends are sutured back together; (2) nerve grafting, required to bridge a gap between nerve ends; and (3) nerve transfer, when the distal or proximal nerve segment is unusable or missing.

Primary Suture Repair

The basic principles of facial nerve repair have changed little since Bunnell performed the first successful infratemporal coaptation in the late 1920s.[15] Primary tension-free neurorrhaphy of fresh nerve endings remains the gold standard. When a sizable gap exists, stretching nerve endings may impair the vascular supply to the nerve.[14] As the nerve is further stretched, the endoneurial connective tissue may rupture. Tension at the repair site also contributes to increases in fibroblastic activity and scarring.[16]

Epineurial repair is generally favored over fascicular repair.[17] Coaptation of the epineurium is easier, faster, and minimizes internal disruption of the nerve and its blood supply.[16] On the other hand, fascicular repairs would potentially provide more precise anatomic reinnervation. Correct fascicle positioning can be confirmed by the continuity of the nerve's surface structures, such as blood vessels (vasa nervorum) within the epineurium.[18]

Lubiatowski describes a technique in which epineurium covering the distal stump is rolled back and a 2-mm nerve segment is resected.[19] An epineural "sleeve" is created over the proximal nerve end and is sutured to the epineurium 2 mm proximal to the coaptation site with 2 sutures (**Fig. 2**). Her study showed faster functional recovery in animals compared with standard epineural end-to-end repair. The epineural sleeve provides

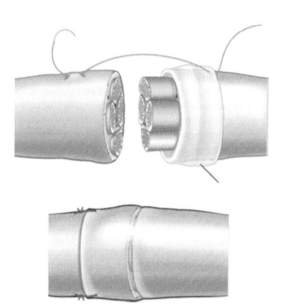

Fig. 2. Diagram of epineural sleeve repair. The free edge of epineurium from the distal stump is rolled back distally and a 2-mm epineural sleeve is created. A 2-mm fragment of distal nerve is resected. Epineural sleeve is pulled over the proximal nerve and is anchored to the epineurium 2 mm proximal to the coaptation site with two 10 to 0 sutures placed 180° apart. (*From* Siemionow M, Brzezicki G. Current techniques and concepts in peripheral nerve repair. Int Rev Neurobiol 2009;87:148; with permission.)

a biological chamber for the axoplasmic fluid leakage from transected nerve ends, providing a favorable environment axonal regeneration. Additionally, this technique provides guidance for regenerating nerve fibers, enabling a higher number of axons to reach target organs and prevents neuroma formation.

Tissue adhesive

The minimum number of 10 to 0 nylon sutures to provide a tension-free coaptation is best to minimize scar formation. However, there are still disadvantages with primary suturing related to foreign body reactions to the suture material, excessive handling and manipulation of the nerve ends, trauma from needle penetration through nerve tissue, and difficulty suturing in confined anatomic locations.[20] Subsequently, alternative techniques have been described in published reports for peripheral nerve repair, including gluing,[21–23] grafting,[24] and laser welding.[25]

Fibrin adhesives (FA) are derived mainly from plasma that facilitates the growth of collagen-producing fibroblasts.[22] Adhesives are easily applied, involve less tissue handling and consequent trauma to the nerve ends, and facilitate the coaptation of the nerve stumps without the demands of microsurgery on both time and surgical expertise.

Knox and colleagues[26] found that the only statistically significant difference between traditional suture neurorrhaphy and FA neural coaptation was the time taken to complete the procedure. Given the reduced operative time required, and ease of application, FA may be an acceptable alternative to suture neurorrhaphy for facial nerve repair.[26]

N-butyl-2-cyanoacrylates used as a tissue adhesive were found to induce fibrosis and foreign body inflammatory reaction and retractile fibrosis, often reducing the nerve diameter up to two-thirds in one study, yet histologic animal studies by another group showed no significant difference in nerve regeneration when comparing suture repair versus cyanoacrylate.[21,27] Starritt and colleagues[28] compared a sutureless method of facial nerve repair using a biodegradable glass fabric with the standard method of microsurgical suture. Both methods of repair were compared with each other and with a normal control group using electrophysiological and morphometric analysis, with the conclusion that glass-wrap entubulation offers an alternative to standard suture repair. The possibility of sutureless neurorrhaphy with biocompatible substances would be ideal, but due to concerns of tensile strength of repair and inflammatory reaction, suture neurorrhaphy remains the gold standard.[29]

Spector and colleagues[30,31] addressed the question whether one should mobilize the nerve extensively to achieve end-to-end repair with a single anastomosis, or eliminate tension by bridging with a nerve graft, leaving the regenerating axons to find their way through 2 anastomoses. They reported rerouting of the nerve to achieve primary coaptation yielded better outcomes compared with bridging the gap with a nerve graft. Gardetto and colleagues[32] reported an anatomic study with bridging up to 15-mm gaps in the facial nerve by removal of the superficial lobe of the parotid gland and mobilizing the branches of the parotid plexus.

Nerve grafts

Millesi[33,34] demonstrated in the 1970s, that grafting of an autogenous nerve segment to bridge a nerve defect leads to better clinical results than suturing the 2 stumps under tension, as is still widely accepted. A nerve graft provides an ideal conduit for regenerating axons because it provides a scaffold that contains Schwann cell basal laminae, and, moreover, these Schwann cells produce growth factors.[35] However, it has several disadvantages, including an extra incision for the removal of a healthy sensory nerve, which will result in a sensory deficit.

The most commonly used donor nerves for facial reanimation include sural nerve, lateral antebrachial cutaneous nerve (LCAN), anterior division of the medial antebrachial cutaneous nerve (MACN), greater auricular nerve, and the motor nerve to the vastus lateralis in cases in which anterolateral thigh free flaps are simultaneously harvested. To choose the best autologous nerve graft, a surgeon has to take into consideration the caliber of the nerve to be repaired, length of the defect, and donor site morbidity.

Does Nerve Graft Polarity Matter?

We are taught that it is important to place a nerve graft so that it is oriented in the same functional direction from which it was harvested. That is, the proximal end of the nerve graft should approximate the proximal end of the host nerve, and the distal end of the graft should anastomose with the distal end of the host nerve, so that axonoplasmic flow should be maintained in the same direction and axons are not lost in branches.[36] However, several animal studies showed that reversing nerve graft polarity of a cable graft did not affect nerve regeneration electrophysiologically or histologically.[37]

Is There a Difference Between Motor Versus Sensory Donor Nerve Graft?

Another interesting question that remains to be answered is whether facial nerve regeneration and synkinesis would differ based on motor versus sensory nerve grafting. In a randomized double-blind placebo-controlled trial using a rat model, motor nerve regeneration increased when nerve gaps were grafted with donor motor nerves in comparison with sensory nerve grafts.[38] MacKinnon postulated that there may be a specificity of motor Schwann cells to produce neurotrophins in response to motor neurites. In another study, MacKinnon found improved regeneration with motor grafting may be a result of the nerve's Schwann cell basal lamina tube size.[14] Motor nerves have larger Schwann cell basal lamina tubes, which may allow more nerve fibers to cross a nerve graft repair. There are occasions in which the opportunity to use a motor nerve, perhaps even vascularized, is possible when anterolateral thigh flap is planned for reconstruction. Future comparisons of patients grafted with motor nerve grafts for facial nerve defects may be possible.

Allografts are nerve grafts harvested from cadavers, which come with the associated risks of immunosuppression.[39] Recently, AxoGen (Burleson, TX, USA) claimed that their allograft named Avance Nerve Graft has no disadvantages related to immunogenicity due to their decellularized and cleansed extracellular matrix. They have an ongoing study, the Ranger Study, with more than 600 nerve repairs enrolled in January 2015.[40]

Non-nervous biological grafts have included artery and vein segments, as well as skeletal muscle autograft. Autogenous vein is an obvious choice of conduit material, owing to its availability, biocompatibility, and ease of harvest. In 1982, Chiu and colleagues[10] presented histologic and electrophysiologic evidence of nerve regeneration through segments of vein used to bridge sciatic nerve gaps in the rat model. The vein walls are resilient enough to act as a barrier against scar ingrowth and have the permeability to allow diffusion of the proper nutrients.[41] They also can provide a mechanical support for the regenerating axonal cone, offering a protected biochemical milieu, away from surrounding tissue.

Nonbiologic Conduits

Because of the unsatisfactory results achieved by the use of natural conduits, attempts were made to develop a better conduit that can support the adhesion, migration, and function of the local cell [42] and can respect as many properties as possible of an ideal nerve conduit, such as[43] the following:

- Biocompatibility
- Biodegradability
- Permeability and porosity
- Protection for axonal growth
- Adequate size
- Adequate flexibility

Along with the development of tissue bioengineering, the past 30 years saw an impressive increase of experimental studies aimed at testing new biomaterials for nerve regeneration, such as decalcified silicone tube, bone tube, nylon fiber tube, and polyurethanes.[41] Most of the conduits the Food and Drug Administration or Conformit Europe approved for clinical use are made of type I collagen, such as NeuraGen, NeuroFlex, and NeuroWrap, but there are also available conduits synthetized of polyglycolic acid and polylactide-caprolactone (Neurotube, Neurolac).[44] The use of a conduit to connect nerve stumps provides an "open" vehicle for modulation of the cellular and molecular environment for nerve regeneration. The addition of Schwann cells, neurotrophic and neurotropic factors can direct the regenerating axons, while the tube protects the nerve from the surrounding tissue.[45] Placing the lacerated ends in each end of a tube instead of trying to match them at the suture site could also leave the axons to find their way more accurately.[46]

Modifications to the common hollow nerve tube have been investigated and include collagen-containing and laminin-containing gels, internal frameworks, supportive cells, growth factors, and conductive polymers.[47,48]

Future perspectives aim in a combined approach to the regenerating process, focusing not only on a scaffold that can support growing axons but also improve Schwann cell migration and deliver growth-promoting factors inside the lumen.[49]

Nerve Substitution

Nerve transfers are indicated when the main trunk of the facial nerve is damaged or unavailable for grafting but the distal nerve branches and mimetic muscles remain viable. Patients with acquired paralysis who have undergone serial clinical and/or electromyographic testing that has failed to show any functional recovery by 6 months should be considered for a reinnervation procedure before significant motor endplate atrophy. There is a general consensus that the best and most predictable results are achieved when neurotization surgery is performed within 2 years of the palsy,[50] although Conley reported success within 4 years of palsy.[51] Increased denervation time and advancing patient age both negatively affect nerve regeneration and may lead to inferior outcomes of reinnervation procedures.

The most common nerve substitution procedures that will be discussed include the hypoglossal, masseteric, and cross-facial sural nerve grafts. There are 3 basic ways in which the nerve transfers are being increasingly used: direct motor neurotization, babysitter and double innervation techniques, and the innervation of neuromuscular transplants.

Hypoglossal–Facial Nerve

Since its introduction by Korte[52] in 1901, the hypoglossal–facial nerve substitution was widely popularized by Conley and Baker.[53] The facial and hypoglossal nerves have a cortical topographic proximity in the motor cortex making the hypoglossal a sensible substitution.[54]

Unfortunately, sacrifice of the hemihypoglossal resulted in unacceptable functional deficits impeding speech and mastication, as well as mass movement and synkinesis of the hemiface (**Fig. 3**).

However, over the past 2 decades, many variations of this procedure have been developed to reduce secondary morbidity. Most notably was partial sacrifice or preservation of the hypoglossal nerve.[55] Animal models have attempted to quantify the degree of hypoglossal axotomy necessary for return of motor function while minimizing tongue atrophy. A rat model demonstrated that 40% hypoglossal axotomy provides a good reinnervation of the orbicularis oculi muscle with minimal tongue atrophy.[56]

In 1991, May and colleagues[55] reported favorable results when using only half of the hypoglossal nerve joined to the extracranial facial nerve by a jump interposition graft. The primary advantage of the interpositional nerve grafting is a satisfactory reinnervation of the facial nerve musculature with less mass movement and synkinesis. Other variations include longitudinal splitting of the hypoglossal nerve to preserve some continuity to the tongue[57] and transposition of the intratemporal facial nerve from the geniculate ganglion for direct end-to-side coaptation without a jump graft.[58]

To date, there are no studies comparing the variations of hypoglossal to facial nerve grafting with standardized outcomes measurements, and so it is difficult to choose which technique is superior. Proponents of the intratemporal facial nerve may argue that stronger neural input is provided by a

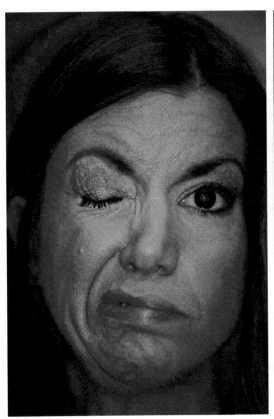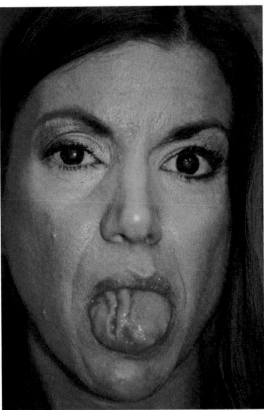

Fig. 3. Patient who underwent end-to-end hypoglossal to facial nerve substitution with sequelae of right facial mass movement and hemi-tongue atrophy. Image on *left* shows right hemifacial mass activation with hypoglossal activation. Image on *right* shows atrophy of the right hemitongue from right hypoglossal nerve sacrifice.

direct end-to-side coaptation without an interposition graft. Others may argue that the process of drilling out the nerve from the mastoid and mobilizing the nerve segment adds mechanical injury and disruption of vascular supply detrimental to regeneration. It is safe to agree that the classical type of hypoglossal–facial nerve repair using the entire proximal hypoglossal nerve should be avoided and that postoperative rehabilitation and neuromuscular retraining are paramount to optimizing facial functional recovery.[59] Neuromuscular retraining is a process of facilitating the return of intended facial movement patterns and eliminating unwanted patterns of facial movement and expression that provide patients with disorders of facial paralysis with the opportunity for the recovery of facial movement and function.[60]

Masseteric to Facial

Masseteric–facial nerve transfer for facial reanimation was initially reported by Spira[61] in 1978 and has recently become popular as a donor nerve in nerve substitution procedures, as well as for neuromuscular transfers. This is evident in numerous recent publications describing surgical anatomy for identification of the masseteric nerve.[62–65]

The masseteric nerve arises from the mandibular division of the trigeminal nerve and leaves the infratemporal fossa through the mandibular notch. It then passes into the masseter muscle from the muscle's medial surface via the space that is formed by the inferior border of the zygomatic arch superiorly and the mandibular notch inferiorly (**Fig. 4**).[64] Next, the nerve generally courses anteroinferiorly along the deep part of the masseter muscle. Therefore, the area that is formed by the inferior border of the zygomatic arch and the mandibular notch can be used as a palpable landmark for identifying the masseteric nerve.[63] A simple way to approach the nerve is at a point 4 cm anterior to the tragus, 1 cm below the zygomatic nerve, and 1.5 cm deep.[66] The fibers of the masseter muscle are separated until the nerve is seen coursing on its undersurface.

Reasons for its increasing popularity include the ease of dissection, adjacent location, sufficient length and caliber, minimal to no donor site morbidity, and rapid functional recovery.[67]

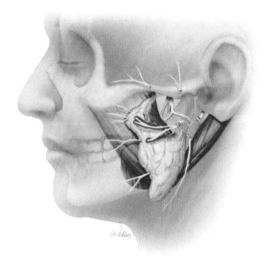

Fig. 4. Drawing depicting surgical anatomy. Microsurgical anastomosis of the descending branch of the masseter nerve to selected buccal branches of the facial nerve is shown. (From Klebuc MJ. Facial reanimation using the masseter-to-facial nerve transfer. Plast Reconstr Surg 2011;127(5):1911; with permission.)

In addition, the physiologic connectedness of the facial and trigeminal nerves has led to trouble-free motor reeducation and the possibility for an effortless smile. Coombs and colleagues[68] found an average of 1542.67 (SD 291.70) myelinated axons in the masseteric nerve compared with the report of Frey and colleagues[69] of 100 to 200 axons at the distal end of a cross-facial nerve graft (CFNG). This represents up to 15 times more axons than found in the distal end of a CFNG. Even in situations in which the contralateral facial nerve is available, the masseteric nerve has been shown to be capable of providing stronger and more reliable innervation of the transferred muscle.[70]

Hontanilla and Marre[71] compared hemihypoglossal nerve versus masseteric nerve in the rehabilitation of short-term facial paralysis and found comparable commissural displacement and contraction velocity between the 2 groups. However, patients undergoing masseteric–facial nerve coaptation showed a significantly faster onset of movement compared with those in the other group (62 days vs 136 days). They concluded that reanimation can be effectively treated by using both methods, but that the use of the masseteric nerve allowed for quicker functional return and avoidance of donor nerve graft morbidity. Thus, they recommend using the masseteric nerve when both techniques are feasible.

Babysitter and Cross-Facial Nerve Grafting

Both the hypoglossal and masseteric nerves are unable to restore spontaneous emotional expression and is the reason why Terzis[72,73] popularized the "babysitter" concept in the 1980s by using a minihypoglossal substitution. The babysitter nerve graft is often used in the setting of CFNG to ensure endogenous growth support by introducing additional sensory or motor (donor) axons into the distal denervated nerve before motor end plate loss as we wait for the axon to traverse the length of the CFNG. The strategy behind the babysitter procedure is that the hypoglossal nerve is used to salvage the paretic facial musculature, but not for reanimation as they are switched out for the cross-facial grafts so that the contralateral facial nerve synchronizes the facial expression (Fig. 5).

Sensory protection, as described by Bain and colleagues,[73] improves functional outcomes. In this approach, the transected end of a sensory nerve is coapted to the end of a transected motor nerve to temporarily innervate denervated muscle before the motor repair, even though no excitable neuromuscular junctions are formed. Ladak and colleagues[74] described another form of "protection" of denervated distal nerve stumps using side-to-side bridges from a healthy donor nerve to improve regeneration without creating a donor nerve deficit. A small number of donor axons regenerating through the side-to-side bridges keep the denervated Schwann cells of the distal nerve stump in a growth-supportive state. Their study aimed to "protect" the pathway of a denervated cross-face nerve graft with end-to-side addition of small adjacent sensory nerves and to subsequently enhance facial nerve motor regeneration through the CFNG.

The fundamental limitation of all of the aforementioned nerve transfer techniques is the inability to achieve spontaneous mimetic motion except CFNG, although the CFNG is still believed to have unpredictable outcomes, and therefore has not completely supplanted hypoglossal/masseter nerve transfers.[70] Split hypoglossal transfers, and more recently masseteric nerve transfers, in conjunction with CFNG provide increased axonal input to the target muscles that may improve results (Fig. 6). One anticipated effect of CFNG is some weakening of facial function on the unaffected side, where compensatory drive would otherwise exacerbate facial asymmetry. Paradoxically, this improves symmetry in most patients and thus is a beneficial outcome.

Yamamoto and colleagues[75] introduced the concept of neural supercharge in recent paralysis and demonstrated the effectiveness of using a hypoglossal input in combination with CFNG to

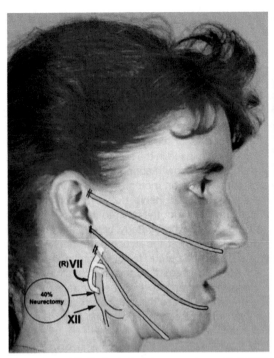 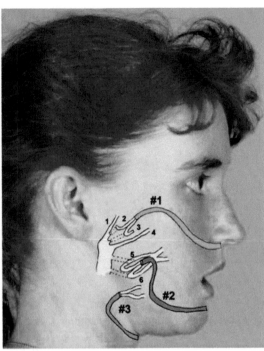

Fig. 5. Stage 1 (*left*): the babysitter procedure with 3 CFNGs and end-to-side coaptation of the facial nerve trunk to the ipsilateral hypoglossal nerve. Stage 2 (*right*): secondary microcoaptations of the CFNGs to the upper zygomatic, main zygomatic, and buccal branches of the right facial nerve. #1#2#3 represent 3 separate cross facial nerve grafts from distal corresponding facial nerve branches from intact facial nerve. (*From* Terzis JK, Tzafetta K. The "babysitter" procedure: minihypoglossal to facial nerve transfer and cross-facial nerve grafting. Plast Reconstr Surg 2009;123(3):872; with permission.)

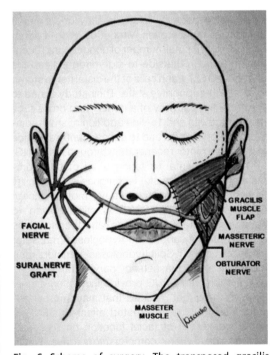

Fig. 6. Scheme of surgery. The transposed gracilis muscle flap is innervated by masseteric nerve (end-to-end anastomosis) and contralateral facial nerve (end-to-side anastomosis) through an interpositional sural nerve graft. (*From* Biglioli F, Colombo V, Tarabbia F, et al. Double innervation in free-flap surgery for long-standing facial paralysis. J Plast Reconstr Aesthet Surg 2012;65:1345; with permission.)

guarantee an adequate quantity of contraction and the correct facial nerve stimulus. Similarly, in case of free-flap transposition, minimization of muscle atrophy should increase functional result, and thus Bianchi[76] proposed masseteric innervation may be helpful in reducing muscle flap atrophy during the denervation period because reanimation starts sooner than when CFNGs are used.[77]

Variations in Nerve Substitution Procedures

In my personal practice, I have incorporated coaptation of the masseteric nerve to distal zygomatic/buccal branch at the Zuker point with simultaneous cable grafting for radical parotid surgery requiring facial nerve sacrifice. I have found clinically that this allows for early reinnervation from the masseteric input as well as a stronger smile, albeit nonmimetic. The close proximity of the masseteric to Zuker point acts as a "babysitter" as we wait for regeneration across the longer cable grafts. Furthermore, by separating input to the zygomaticus from the cable grafting there is theoretically less synkinesis. Video 1 shows photos and video of a patient 2 months after facial nerve sacrifice for which I performed cable grafting with multiple branches of the MACN and a separate masseteric nerve to distal buccal branch coaptation (see Video 1; available online at http://www.facialplastic.theclinics.com/). I have found there is essentially no added morbidity and minimal surgical time added, as operative exposure is provided with extirpation. At 2 months, he shows facial muscle movement with masseteric nerve activation. His resting tone is still diminished, but improves as there is recovery from the cable grafting as seen in his 1-year postoperative video (Video 2; available online at http://www.facialplastic.theclinics.com/). The photographs in **Fig. 7** show another patient who recovers good excursion and resting tone with less synkinesis in cable grafting of facial nerve with simultaneous masseteric to distal buccal branch nerve substitution.

The recent popularity of the masseteric nerve substitution over the hypoglossal nerve substitution is attributed to stronger axonal input and quicker recovery time.[78] Although I have found this to be true in my practice, I have also observed that my patients with masseteric input do not recover the resting tone that I see in my patients with hypoglossal input. The study by Hontanilla and Marre[71] comparing masseteric versus hypoglossal nerve substitution did not note any difference in resting tone and favored masseteric as a stronger input. I attribute the observed differences in my clinical practice to the characteristics of the muscle use and function. The tongue is in a constant dynamic state and perhaps has a higher resting tone than the masseter muscle, which is a demand muscle called on during mastication. **Figs. 8** and **9** show patients who underwent

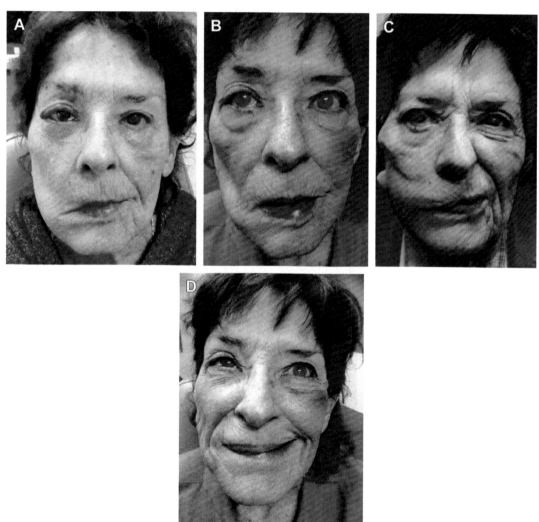

Fig. 7. Patients after simultaneous masseteric to buccal and cable nerve grafts to facial nerve after radical resection of parotid and facial nerve for malignancy. Photos show significant resting and smile asymmetry immediately postoperatively and some functional recovery at 1 year. (*A*) Shows patient immediately postop at rest with right facial paralysis. She has her lower lid taped for support. (*B*) The patient at rest with recovery of right facial tone at one year from cable grafting of the facial nerve. (*C*) Shows patient with right facial paralysis immediately postoperative with attempted smile. (*D*) Shows patient with smile and activation of masseteric nerve with clenching.

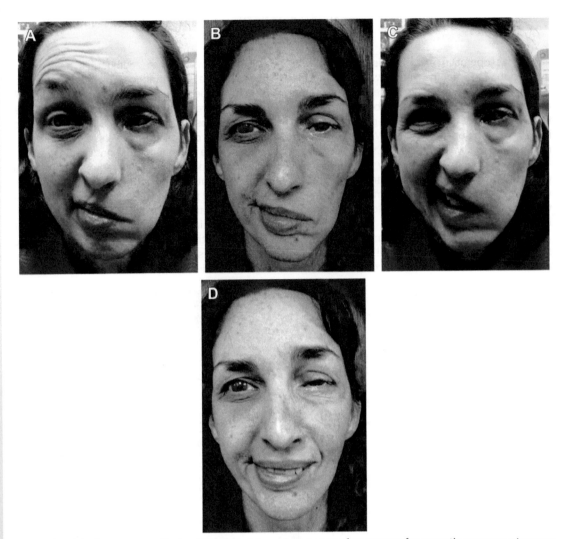

Fig. 8. (*A*, *B*) Patient preoperatively with left facial paralysis 1 year after surgery for acoustic neuroma at repose (*A*) and with smiling (*B*). (*C*, *D*) Patient 1 year postoperatively from masseteric to facial nerve substitution procedure at repose (*C*) and with clenching (*D*). Note diminished resting symmetry.

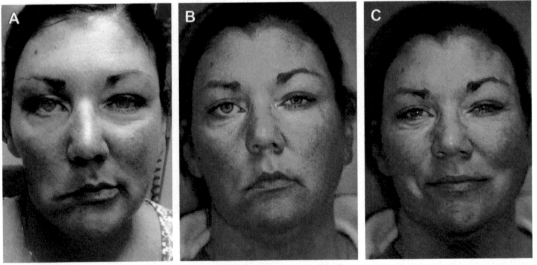

Fig. 9. (*A*) Patient with right facial paralysis 15 months after cerebral aneurysm. (*B*) Patient 24 months after masseteric to facial nerve substitution in repose still with diminished resting tone as noted with scleral show and effacement of the nasolabial fold. (*C*) Patient with right facial activation on clenching at 24 months postoperative.

masseteric to facial nerve main trunk substitution who exhibit very good excursion with clenching and masseter activation, but poor static tone in repose or speaking. **Fig. 10** and Videos 3 and 4 show patients with good resting tone and perhaps not as notable excursion (see Videos 3 and 4; available online at http://www.facialplastic.theclinics.com/). A study to compare the 2 groups with standard outcome measures will be illustrative.

EMERGING TECHNOLOGIES

Advances in tissue engineering and nerve regeneration, including novel regenerative conduits, neuromuscular interfaces, bionics, and artificial muscle, hold promise in facial reanimation.

Most bioengineered interface strategies rely on reanimating intact neuromuscular systems. In some patients, the muscle or nerve tissue is no longer viable for recording or stimulation. Electroactive polymer artificial muscle was developed in the 1990s (SRI International) for several robotic applications. Artificial muscle products function by converting electrical force to mechanical motion.[79,80]

There are animal studies of an implantable system for restoration of eye blink in hemiparalysis patients in which the device records electromyographic signals from a small electrode implanted in the orbicularis oculi muscle on the healthy side of the face.[81] The signals picked up are delivered as electrical impulses via electrodes to the corresponding muscles on the contralateral side. There is potential to create a multielectrode device for other facial muscles.[82]

Mesenchymal stem cells (MSCs) are an attractive cell source for the regeneration of nerve tissue, as they are able to self-renew and differentiate into diverse cell types. MSCs contain neurotrophic factors that are known as the other regeneration component of nerves. Some reports have described the possibilities of MSCs on peripheral nerve regeneration.

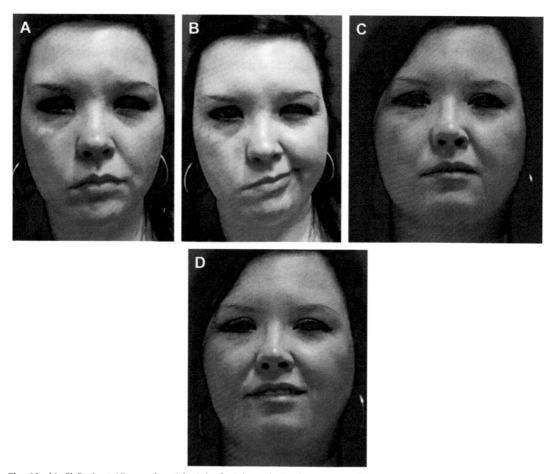

Fig. 10. (*A, B*) Patient 15 months with right facial paralysis after surgery for cavernous hemangioma of the pons at rest (*A*) and smiling (*B*). (*C, D*) Patient 1 year after hemihypoglossal to facial nerve main trunk at rest (*C*, note improved resting tone) and with tongue activation (*D*).

Despite advances in the medical and surgical management of facial nerve injuries, functional recovery is often poor, particularly after a complete transection. Approaches for restoring function include a variety of surgical approaches, as there is no defined algorithm. The options depend on the individual patient factors, status of the facial nerve, and surgeon ability. The evolution of surgical technique, collaborations with biomedical engineers, and new technology may hold promise for improving the treatment of these patients.

SUPPLEMENTARY DATA

Supplementary data related to this article can be found online at http://dx.doi.org/10.1016/j.fsc.2015.09.006.

REFERENCES

1. Lundborg G. Nerve injury and repair: regeneration, reconstruction, and cortical remodeling. 2nd edition. Philadelphia: Churchill Livingstone; 2005.
2. Lee SK, Wolfe SW. Peripheral nerve injury and repair. J Am Acad Orthop Surg 2000;8(4):243–52.
3. Gordon T, Tyreman N, Raji MA. The basis for diminished functional recovery after delayed peripheral nerve repair. J Neurosci 2011;31:5325–34.
4. Geuna S, Raimondo S, Ronchi G, et al. Chapter 3: histology of the peripheral nerve and changes occurring during nerve regeneration. Int Rev Neurobiol 2009;87:27–46.
5. Fu S, Gordon T. The cellular and molecular basis of peripheral nerve regeneration. Mol Neurobiol 1997; 14:67–116.
6. Terenghi G. Peripheral nerve regeneration and neurotrophic factors. J Anat 1999;194:1–14.
7. Muir D. The potentiation of peripheral nerve sheaths in regeneration and repair. Exp Neurol 2010;233: 102–11.
8. Seddon JJ, Medawar PB, Smith H. Rate of regeneration of peripheral nerves in man. J Physiol 1943; 102:191–215.
9. Rodriguez FJ, Verdu E, Ceballos D. Nerve guides seeded with autologous Schwann cells improve nerve regeneration. Exp Neurol 2000;161(2):571–84.
10. Chiu DT, Janecka I, Krizek TJ. Autogenous vein graft as a conduit for nerve regeneration. Surgery 1982; 91:226–33.
11. Aebischer P, Salessiotis AN, Winn SR. Basic fibroblast growth factor released from synthetic guidance channels facilitates peripheral nerve regeneration across long nerve gaps. J Neurosci Res 1989;23:282–9.
12. Madison R, da Silva CF, Dikkes P. Increased rate of peripheral nerve regeneration using bioresorbable nerve guides and a laminin-containing gel. Exp Neurol 1985;88:767–72.
13. Terzis JK, Smith KL. The peripheral nerve. Structure, function, reconstruction. New York: Raven Press; 1990. p. 127.
14. Moradzadeh A, Borschel GH, Luciano JP, et al. The impact of motor and sensory nerve architecture on nerve regeneration. Exp Neurol 2008;212:370–6.
15. Bunnell S. Surgical repair of the facial nerve. Arch Otolaryngol 1937;25:235–59.
16. Matsuyama T, Mackay M, Midha R. Peripheral nerve repair and grafting techniques: a review. Neurol Med Chir (Tokyo) 2000;40:187–99.
17. Dvali L, Mackinnon S. Nerve repair, grafting, and nerve transfers. Clin Plast Surg 2003;30:203–21.
18. Wilgis EFS. Techniques of epineural and group fascicular repair. In: Gelberman RH, editor. Operative nerve repair and reconstruction, vol. 1. Philadelphia: JB Lippincott; 1991. p. 287–93.
19. Lubiatowski P, Unsal FM, Nair D, et al. The epineural sleeve technique for nerve graft reconstruction enhances nerve recovery. Microsurgery 2008;28: 160–7.
20. Levinthal R, Brown WJ, Rand RW. Comparison of fascicular, interfascicular and epineural suture techniques in the repair of simple nerve lacerations. J Neurosurg 1977;47(5):744–50.
21. Gencer ZK, Ozkiris M, Saydam L, et al. The comparison of histological results of experimentally created facial nerve defects repaired by 2 different anastomosis techniques: classic suture technique or tissue adhesives for nerve anastomosis? J Craniofac Surg 2014;25(2):652–6.
22. Sameem M, Wood TJ, Bain JR. A systematic review on the use of fibrin glue for peripheral nerve repair. Plast Reconstr Surg 2011;127:2381–90.
23. Bento RF, Miniti A. Comparison between fibrin tissue adhesive, epineural suture and natural union in intratemporal facial nerve of cats. Acta Otolaryngol Suppl 1989;465:1–36.
24. Evans G. Peripheral nerve injury: a review and approach to tissue engineered constructs. Anat Rec 2001;263:396–404.
25. Happak W, Neumayer C, Holak G, et al. Morphometric and functional results after CO(2) laser welding of nerve coaptations. Lasers Surg Med 2000; 27(1):66–72.
26. Knox CJ, Hohman MH, Kleiss IJ, et al. Facial nerve repair: fibrin adhesive coaptation versus epineurial suture repair in a rodent model. Laryngoscope 2013;123:1618–21.
27. Choi BH, Kim BY, Huh JY, et al. Microneural anastomosis using cyanoacrylate adhesives. Int J Oral Maxillofac Surg 2004;33(8):777–80.
28. Starritt NE, Kettle SA, Glasby MA. Sutureless repair of the facial nerve using biodegradable glass fabric. Laryngoscope 2011;121(8):1614–9.

29. Siemionow M, Brzezicki G. Current techniques and concepts in peripheral nerve repair. Int Rev Neurobiol 2009;87:141–72.

30. Spector JG, Lee P, Perterein J, et al. Facial nerve regeneration through autologous nerve grafts: a clinical and experimental study. Laryngoscope 1991; 101:537–54.

31. Spector JG. Neural repair in facial paralysis: clinical and experimental studies. Eur Arch Otorhinolaryngol 1997;254:68–75.

32. Gardetto A, Kovacs P, Piegger J, et al. Direct coaptation of extensive facial nerve defects after removal of the superficial part of the parotid gland: an anatomic study. Head Neck 2002;24:1047–53.

33. Millesi H. Nerve suture and grafting to restore the extratemporal facial nerve. Clin Plast Surg 1979;6: 333–41.

34. Millesi H. Nerve grafting. Clin Plast Surg 1984;11: 105–13.

35. Lundborg G. Alternatives to autologous nerve grafts. Handchir Mikrochir Plast Chir 2004;36(1):1–7.

36. Sotereanos DG, Seaber AV, Urbaniak JR, et al. Reversing nerve-graft polarity in a rat model: the effect on function. J Reconstr Microsurg 1992;8(4): 303–7.

37. Nakatsuka H, Takamatsu K, Koshimune M, et al. Experimental study of polarity in reversing cable nerve grafts. J Reconstr Microsurg 2002;18(6): 509–15.

38. Nichols CM, Brenner MJ, Fox IK, et al. Effects of motor versus sensory nerve grafts on peripheral nerve regeneration. Exp Neurol 2004;190:347–55.

39. Sedaghati T, Jell G, Seifalian AM. Regenerative medicine applications in organ transplantation. In: Orlando G, editor. Nerve regeneration and bioengineering. Elsevier; 2013. p. 799–810.

40. Safa B, Weber RV, Rinker B, et al. Impact of age on outcomes in peripheral nerve repair with processed nerve allograft. ASPN 2015 Annual Meeting, Paradise Islands, Bahamas.

41. Battiston B, Geuna S, Ferrero M, et al. Nerve repair by means of tubulization: literature review and personal clinical experience comparing biological and synthetic conduits for sensory nerve repair. Microsurgery 2005;25(4):258–67.

42. Gu X, Ding F, Williams DF. Neural tissue engineering options for peripheral nerve regeneration. Biomaterials 2014;35:6143–56.

43. de Ruiter GC, Malessy MJ, Yaszemski MJ, et al. Designing ideal conduits for peripheral nerve repair. Neurosurg Focus 2009;26:E5.

44. Pabari A, Lloyd-Hughes H, Seifalian AM, et al. Nerve conduits for peripheral nerve surgery. Plast Reconstr Surg 2014;133:1420–30.

45. Battiston B, Raimondo S, Tos P, et al. Chapter 11: tissue engineering of peripheral nerves. Int Rev Neurobiol 2009;87:227–49.

46. Ljungberg C, Johansson-Ruden G, Boström KJ, et al. Neuronal survival using a resorbable synthetic conduit as an alternative to primary nerve repair. Microsurgery 1999;19(6):259–64.

47. Zhang BG, Quigley AF, Myers DE, et al. Recent advances in nerve tissue engineering. Int J Artif Organs 2014;37:277–91.

48. Nectow AR, Marra KG, Kaplan DL. Biomaterials for the development of peripheral nerve guidance conduits. Tissue Eng Part B Rev 2012;18:40–50.

49. Chang WC, Hawkes E, Keller CG, et al. Axon repair: surgical application at a subcellular scale. Wiley Interdiscip Rev Nanomed Nanobiotechnol 2012;2:151–61.

50. Bascom DA, Schaitkin BM, May M, et al. Facial nerve repair: a retrospective review. Facial Plast Surg 2000;16:309–13.

51. Conley J. The treatment of long-standing facial paralysis: a new concept. Trans Am Acad Ophthalmol Otolaryngol 1975;78:386–92.

52. Korte W. Ein Fall von Nervenpfropfung: des Nervus facialis auf den Nervus hypoglossus. Dtsch Med Wochenschr 1903;17:293Y5.

53. Conley J, Baker DC. Hypoglossal–facial nerve anastomosis for reinnervation of the paralyzed face. Plast Reconstr Surg 1979;63:63–72.

54. Hammerschlag PE. Facial reanimation with jump interpositional graft hypoglossal facial anastomosis and hypoglossal facial anastomosis: evolution in management of facial paralysis. Laryngoscope 1999;109:1–23.

55. May M, Sobol SM, Mester SJ. Hypoglossal-facial nerve interpositional-jump graft for facial reanimation without tongue atrophy. Otolaryngol Head Neck Surg 1991;104:818Y25.

56. Kalantarian B, Rice DC, Tiangco DA, et al. Gains and losses of the XII–VII component of the "babysitter" procedure: a morphometric analysis. J Reconstr Microsurg 1998;14:459–71.

57. Cusimano MD, Sekhar L. Partial hypoglossal to facial nerve anastomosis for reinnervation of the paralyzed face in patients with lower cranial nerve palsies: technical note. Neurosurgery 1994;35(3):532–3.

58. Slattery WH 3rd, Cassis AM, Wilkinson EP, et al. Side-to-end hypoglossal to facial anastomosis with transposition of the intratemporal facial nerve. Otol Neurotol 2014;35(3):509–13.

59. Lindsay RW, Robinson M, Hadlock TA. Comprehensive facial rehabilitation improves function in people with facial paralysis: a 5-year experience at the Massachusetts Eye and Ear Infirmary. Phys Ther 2010; 90:391–7.

60. Vanswearingen J. Facial rehabilitation: a neuromuscular reeducation, patient-centered approach. Facial Plast Surg 2008;24(2):250–9.

61. Spira M. Anastomosis of masseteric nerve to lower division of facial nerve for correction of lower facial paralysis. Plast Reconstr Surg 1978;61:330–4.

62. Borschel GH, Kawamura DH, Kasukurthi R, et al. The motor nerve to the masseter muscle: an anatomic and histomorphometric study to facilitate its use in facial reanimation. J Plast Reconstr Aesthet Surg 2012;65(3):363–6.

63. Cotrufo S, Hart A, Payne AP, et al. Topographic anatomy of the nerve to masseter: an anatomical and clinical study. J Plast Reconstr Aesthet Surg 2011; 64:1424–9.

64. Fournier HD, Denis F, Papon X, et al. An anatomical study of the motor distribution of the mandibular nerve for a masseteric–facial anastomosis to restore facial function. Surg Radiol Anat 1997;19: 241–4.

65. Collar RM, Byrne PJ, Boahene KD. The subzygomatic triangle: rapid, minimally invasive identification of the masseteric nerve for facial reanimation. Plast Reconstr Surg 2013;132:183–8.

66. Hontanilla B, Qiu SS. Transposition of the hemimasseteric muscle for dynamic rehabilitation of facial paralysis. J Craniofac Surg 2012;23: 203–5.

67. Brenner E, Schoeller T. Masseteric nerve: a possible donor for facial nerve anastomosis? Clin Anat 1998; 11:396–400.

68. Coombs CJ, Ek EW, Wu T, et al. Masseteric–facial nerve coaptation—an alternative technique for facial nerve reinnervation. J Plast Reconstr Aesthet Surg 2009;62:1580–8.

69. Frey M, Happak W, Girsch W, et al. Histomorphometric studies in patients with facial palsy treated by functional muscle transplantation: new aspects for the surgical concept. Ann Plast Surg 1991;26: 370e9.

70. Bae Y, Zuker RM, Manktelow RT, et al. A comparison of commissure excursion following gracilis muscle transplantation for facial paralysis using a cross-face nerve graft versus the motor nerve to the masseter nerve. Plast Reconstr Surg 2006;117(7): 2407–13.

71. Hontanilla B, Marre D. Comparison of hemihypoglossal nerve versus masseteric nerve transpositions in the rehabilitation of short-term facial paralysis using the Facial Clima evaluating system. Plast Reconstr Surg 2012;130:662e–72e.

72. Terzis JK. 'Babysitters': an exciting new concept in facial reanimation. The facial nerve. In: Castro D, editor. Proceedings of the Sixth International Symposium on the Facial Nerve. Rio de Janeiro (Brazil): 1988.

73. Bain JR, Hason Y, Veltri KL, et al. Clinical application of sensory protection of denervated muscle: case report. J Neurosurg 2008;109:955–61.

74. Ladak A, Schembri P, Olson J, et al. Side-to-side nerve grafts sustain chronically denervated peripheral nerve pathways during axon regeneration and result in improved functional reinnervation. Neurosurgery 2011;68:1654–65.

75. Yamamoto Y, Sekido M, Furukawa H, et al. Surgical rehabilitation of reversible facial palsy: facial-hypoglossal network system based on neural signal augmentation/neural supercharge concept. J Plast Reconstr Aesthet Surg 2007;60(3):223–31.

76. Bianchi B, Ferri A, Ferrari S, et al. The masseteric nerve: a versatile power source in facial animation techniques. British Journal of Oral and Maxillofacial Surgery 2014;52(3):264–9.

77. Biglioli F, Colombo V, Tarabbia F, et al. Double innervation in free-flap surgery for long-standing facial paralysis. J Plast Reconstr Aesthet Surg 2012;65:1345.

78. Klebuc MJ. Facial reanimation using the masseter-to-facial nerve transfer. Plast Reconstr Surg 2011; 127(5):1909–15.

79. Tollefson TT, Senders CW. Restoration of eyelid closure in facial paralysis using artificial muscle: preliminary cadaveric analysis. Laryngoscope 2007;117:1907–11.

80. Senders CW, Tollefson TT, Curtiss S, et al. Force requirements for artificial muscle to create an eyelid blink with eyelid sling. Arch Facial Plast Surg 2010; 12:30–6.

81. McDonnall D, Guillory KS. Gossman MD. Restoration of blink in facial paralysis patients using FES. In: NER '09. 4th International IEEE/EMBS Conference on Neural Engineering. 2009. p. 76–9.

82. McDonnall D, Askin R, Smith C, et al. Verification and validation of an electrode array for a blink prosthesis for facial paralysis patients. In: 6th International IEEE/EMBS Conference on Neural Engineering (NER). 2013. p. 1167–70.

Index

Note: Page numbers of article titles are in **boldface** type.

A

Allograft(s)
  in static rehabilitation of paralyzed midface, 31
Antiviral agents
  in Bell's palsy management, 7
Autologous tissue grafts
  in static rehabilitation of paralyzed midface, 30

B

Bell's palsy, **1–10**
  anatomy of facial nerve in, 1–2
  causes of, 2
  diagnosis of, 2–6
    facial assessment in, 3
  differential diagnosis of, 4
  incidence of, 2
  introduction, 1
  management of, 6–8
    antiviral agents in, 7
    corticosteroids in, 6–7
    long-term, 8
    outcomes of, 7
    physical therapy in, 7
    surgical decompression in, 6
    synkinesis following, 8
Botulinum toxin
  in facial paralysis management, **11–20**
    contralateral normal side
      asymmetry-related, 17
    future directions in, 18
    introduction, 11–12
    neuromodulator injection with, 15–16
    NMR with, 13–15
    options in, 13–17
    patient evaluation prior to, 12–13
    risks associated with, 17

C

Corticosteroid(s)
  in Bell's palsy management, 6–7

E

Eye(s)
  in facial paralysis
    assessment of, 22–23

management of, **21–28**
  anatomy related to, 23–25
  introduction, 21–22
  lower eyelid tightening, 26–27
  operative technique, 25
  surgical indications, 23
  upper eyelid loading, 25–26
Eyelid(s)
  lower
    tightening of
      in facial paralysis management, 26–27
  upper
    loading
      in facial paralysis management, 25–26

F

Facial nerve
  anatomy of, 1–2
Facial paralysis, **1–10**. *See also* Bell's palsy
  consequences of, 21–22
  correction of, **29–35**
    alternative therapies in, 17–18
    botulinum toxin in, **11–20** (*See also* Botulinum toxin, in facial paralysis management)
    eye management in, **21–28** (*See also* Eye(s), in facial paralysis, management of)
    future directions in, 18
    gracilis free flap in, **47–60** (*See also* Gracilis free flap)
    introduction, 29–30
    midface
      static rehabilitation, 30–31
    nerve repair in, 72–81 (*See also* Facial reanimation, components of)
    sternohyoid flap in, **61–69** (*See also* Sternohyoid flap, for facial reanimation)
    surgical techniques in, **29–35**
      introduction, 29–30
      percutaneous suture–based slings, 32–34
      rhytidectomy, 31
      static suspension sling, 31–32
  differential diagnosis of, 4
  introduction, 1
  nerve anatomy related to, 72
  nerve injury process in, 71–72
  smile restoration after

Facial Plast Surg Clin N Am 24 (2016) 85–87
http://dx.doi.org/10.1016/S1064-7406(15)00123-6
1064-7406/16/$ – see front matter © 2016 Elsevier Inc. All rights reserved.

Moving?

Make sure your subscription moves with you!

To notify us of your new address, find your **Clinics Account Number** (located on your mailing label above your name), and contact customer service at:

Email: journalscustomerservice-usa@elsevier.com

800-654-2452 (subscribers in the U.S. & Canada)
314-447-8871 (subscribers outside of the U.S. & Canada)

Fax number: 314-447-8029

Elsevier Health Sciences Division
Subscription Customer Service
3251 Riverport Lane
Maryland Heights, MO 63043

*To ensure uninterrupted delivery of your subscription, please notify us at least 4 weeks in advance of move.

ELSEVIER